HOMEOPATHY
in Primary Care

For Churchill Livingstone:

Commissioning editor: Inta Ozols
Project manager: Valerie Burgess
Project development editor: Mairi McCubbin
Design direction: Judith Wright
Project controller: Pat Miller
Copy editor: Holly Regan-Jones
Indexer: Tarrant Ranger Indexing Agency
Sales promotion executive: Hilary Brown

HOMEOPATHY
in Primary Care

BOB LECKRIDGE BSc MB ChB MFHom
Specialist in Homoeopathic Medicine, Glasgow Homoeopathic Hospital;
Director of Education, Academic Departments,
Glasgow Homoeopathic Hospital, Glasgow, UK

Forewords by

DAVID REILLY FRCP MRCGP FFHom
Director, Academic Departments and Lead Consultant Physician,
Glasgow Homoeopathic Hospital, Glasgow;
Honorary Senior Lecturer in Medicine,
University Department of Medicine, the Royal Infirmary,
Glasow, UK

JONATHAN SHORE MBChB MD MFHom DHt
Hahnemann Medical Clinic, Albany,
California, USA

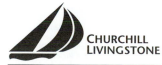

CHURCHILL LIVINGSTONE

NEW YORK EDINBURGH LONDON MADRID MELBOURNE SAN FRANCISCO TOKYO 1997

CHURCHILL LIVINGSTONE
Medical Division of Pearson Professional Limited

Distributed in the United States of America by Churchill Livingstone, 650 Avenue of the Americas, New York, N.Y. 10011, and by associated companies, branches and representatives throughout the world.

© Pearson Professional Limited 1997

First published 1997

ISBN 0 443 05521 1

British Library Cataloguing in Publication Data
A catalogue record of this book is available from the British Library.

Library of Congress Cataloging in Publication Data
A catalog record for this book is available from the Library of Congress.

Note
Medical knowledge is constantly changing. As new information becomes available, changes in treatment, procedures, equipment and the use of drugs become necessary. The author and the publishers have, as far as it is possible, taken care to ensure that the information given in this text is accurate and up to date. However, readers are strongly advised to confirm that the information, especially with regard to drug usage, complies with latest legislation and standards of practice.

The
publisher's
policy is to use
paper manufactured
from sustainable forests

Produced by Longman Singapore Publishers (Pte) Ltd
Printed in Singapore

CONTENTS

*Allergies – anal fissure – anger – chickenpox – chilblains – colic –
fears and phobias – gall bladder colic – glandular fever – grief –
impotence – infant snuffles – infertility – influenza – injuries –
intermittent claudication – mastalgia – measles – mumps –
nightmares/night terrors – premenstrual syndrome – recurrent
catarrhal complaints – teething problems – tinnitus – urethral
syndrome – warts*

FOREWORD
DAVID REILLY

Would homeopathy help? As a primary care worker, your patients have asked you this, or, if they have not, the signs are they shortly will. As a carer, you may even by now be one step ahead of the patient in wondering if there might be another approach to help the person better, or maybe avoid side effects, addiction or high costs. As a potential patient, or concerned family member yourself, you can see the issues from both sides of the fence. Most of all, you do not want to place your patient at risk, or turn your back on the core skills and benefits of contemporary medicine. This has given you the valued gift of caution and a wariness of dabbling. How do you test the waters while avoiding the sharks?

This book will help you safely examine this area and find answers to the following questions. What is homeopathy, does it work, when, and for whom? Is there any point in referring on to a specialist, and how will their approach converge or differ from your own? Are there any simple things you could learn, or recommend directly yourself? How do you begin to study the subject and how do you go a bit further in your understanding? Should you go on that course?

You do not need to want to use homeopathy to benefit from it, or this book. The insights and different perspectives will enrich your daily work and care. If that is what you seek from this book you will want to scan, but not study Chapters 5–8 on chronic case management and repertorisation, get a feel for the clinical scope of the discipline in the cases and references sections (Sections 3 and 4), and learn from the common questions in Section 2. Still, I would urge you to at least try one or two simple first aid applications. The students on the Foundations of Homoeopathy course in Glasgow, with which this book dovetails, begin with Arnica in bruising injuries, Chamomilla in teething babies and Colocynthus in infant colic. In this book, you will find what you need to apply these remedies confidently and safely in your practice (and so at least catch up with the mothers in your practice who are already buying it over-the-counter!).

You will also find this book of real value if you have decided to become a student, either at first year level (perhaps to the UK Faculty of Homoeopathy's Primary Care Certificate level), or beyond that, towards more specialist levels of knowledge and qualification.

You can have confidence in the author's work. He has been a general practitioner for 15 years, and to his skills as a humane and balanced doctor, he has integrated 10 years of homeopathic study and practice. He has made his way from where you now are – be it as a novice or student, through to a specialist, but also importantly, he has been a teacher for 8 years with the Academic Departments of Glasgow Homoeopathic Hospital, learning from our students what the educational needs are, of today's conventional primary care workers. He has developed a well-deserved reputation for his personal qualities and his skill and I have very much enjoyed working with him.

Over 20% of Scotland's general practitioners have completed Foundation training in homeopathy through the Glasgow model, learning in an interdisciplinary way, with nurses, dentists, midwives, pharmacists, veterinary surgeons and other paramedical professions. Together they have pioneered the exploration of where and how this additional therapeutic approach can enrich the conventional approach to patients, while improving on their therapy. Research has shown that they are more than satisfied with the results (Reilly 1995). But if you should decide to join them, under the skilled guidance of this book, beware – you will discover that there is more in medical heaven and earth than was taught in your medical training. Enjoy your new adventure.

1997   D. R.

Reference
Reilly DT. 1995 Clarifying competence by defining its limits. Lessons from the Glasgow Education Model of Homoeopathic Training. Complementary Therapies in Medicine 3: 21–24

Further information on the Glasgow Model and linked courses can be obtained from ADHom: The Academic Departments of Glasgow Homoeopathic Hospital, 1000 Great Western Road, Glasgow G12 0NR, UK. Tel: +44 141 337 1824. Fax +44 141 211 1610.

FOREWORD
JONATHAN SHORE

Homeopathy in Primary Care is an excellent work which amply fulfills its stated purpose of introducing basic homeopathic knowledge in such a way that it can be clearly grasped and put to a practical test in the conditions of everyday medical practice.

It is no small accomplishment to present a subtle and complex technique in such a simple and immediately practical fashion as to enable its successful application, whilst simultaneously allowing the true beauty and depth of possibility inherent in the system to shine through. This is, in fact, the signature of someone who has a wisdom distilled from many years of conscientious practice; who has faced and worked through the very problems this book addresses.

Anyone who takes the trouble to study and digest the information presented here, will not fail to accumulate enough successful prescriptions to satisfy themselves of the fact that homeopathic medicines have a truly remarkable action – remarkable from a number of points of view. It is evident to all who have investigated the subject with an open mind that, despite all theoretical denials of the possibility of action, these preparations do, in fact, have a definite action on the human organism. What is even more remarkable, however, for those concerned with the long-term health of their fellow beings, is the scope of this action. It appears not only to palliate symptoms and block their expression, while the chronic process of tissue destruction advances, but, in a significant number of cases, to remove the underlying disease process itself. This simultaneous cure and prevention, and the speed and elegance with which they occur, bestow an experience on both patient and prescriber which is unforgettable.

There is, however, another level, another depth, to this text which I feel needs to be brought out. The quote on page 4 (repeated again here) from the British Medical Association's 1993 publication opens the question:

One of the main reasons for the current upsurge of official interest in non-conventional medicine is the rapidly increasing number of patients who are seeking help from such practitioners. This has prompted the Council of Europe to state 'It is not possible to consider this phenomenon as a medical side-issue. It must reflect a genuine public need which is in urgent need of definition and analysis'.

The reasons for this phenomenon are complex, but I feel it is safe to say that, in part, it results from the failure of modern biological science to grant full citizenship to one of the prime facets of human experience, that of the emotions or feelings. These powerful and mysteriously acting influences which constitute the field of relationship between practitioner and patient, have been very gradually, yet almost entirely, excluded from the process of treatment. One of the, as yet, unappreciated gifts of homeopathy is the reintroduction of the possibility of relationship. A relationship which arises from the form, rather than the intent, of the system. This aspect of homeopathic practice is beautifully brought out in the author's writing. Its spirit illuminates the text in such a fashion that an honest and conscientious study of the deceptively simple principles and suggestions contained in the first 70 pages would greatly increase the healing capacity of any practitioner, even if they never prescribed a homeopathic remedy.

1996   J. S.

PREFACE

On reflection, there are two main reasons for writing this book. The first is to enhance primary care medicine and the second is to enhance the practice of homeopathy.

For most of my life my goal was to become a doctor, or, more specifically, a family doctor. I was, therefore, quite surprised to find, on reaching my goal (becoming a family doctor in a small village in southern Scotland), that being a family doctor was frequently not very satisfying because it was largely not about healing. My discovery of the therapeutic potential of homeopathy enabled me to find a way of practising a kind of medicine which was more in touch with 'healing'. I found that integrating homeopathy into primary care medicine was not always easy but was enormously rewarding and made a significant difference to patients' lives.

Within a few years of learning the subject, I was drawn into teaching it to others. The courses run in Glasgow by Dr David Reilly were my first contact with homeopathy and it was he who encouraged me to join the teaching team. Our courses teach homeopathy only to health care professionals, the vast majority of whom are working in primary care. Time and again, I would find myself answering the same questions and helping students with the same difficulties. I realised that there were no books available which focused on primary care workers and which answered their particular problems, so I decided to write one myself.

Homeopathy, as a therapeutic modality, originated in primary care (although it was not called that 200 years ago); however, in the 20th century it seems to have lost touch with its roots. Too often now, desk-based homeopathy is thought of as 'real homeopathy'. Patients typically suffer from chronic diseases and the homeopathic process focuses almost exclusively on a lengthy examination of the patient's mental state. Whilst such homeopathic practice is valuable, I fear the tail has begun to wag the dog. The emphasis of this book is squarely on primary care homeopathy and, I hope, as such, it will contribute to the development of homeopathy as a therapy.

I hope this book will help health care professionals to conduct their work more effectively and to enable them to enjoy the therapeutic, healing potential of this therapy. I also hope this book will remind homeopaths of their origins and help to stimulate homeopathic teachers and practitioners to find ways to develop effective, safe, clinical homeopathy.

1996   B.L.

ACKNOWLEDGEMENTS

Many people have helped and inspired me along the road to becoming a homeopathic specialist. I would particularly like to acknowledge four of my contemporaries, without whom I would not be where I am today. All four of these colleagues have also become my good friends.

First and foremost, Dr David Reilly of Glasgow whose convincing and charismatic teaching first introduced me to the subject back in 1984. David has become a great friend since those days and we now work together at the Glasgow Homoeopathic Hospital as clinicians and as directors of the extremely popular teaching programme which is being run in several other countries besides Scotland.

Dr Jonathon Shore of Mill Valley, California, was an early inspiration and introduced me to the 'Vithoulkas' revolution which has rejuvenated 20th century homeopathy.

Dr Massimo Mangialavori of Modena, Italy, has delighted many with his warm, humble personality and has inspired many of us with his clear presentations of the themes of remedies and the concept of 'families' of remedies.

Dr Jan Scholten of Utrecht, The Netherlands, has similarly delighted audiences with his warm personality and his inspired analysis of remedies and their relationships within the periodic table.

There are many others who have inspired me and who have become good friends and colleagues. I also owe a debt of gratitude to the authors of the books I have used for my own personal study over the years – from Samuel Hahnemann to Hamish Boyd.

BACKGROUND AND CLINICAL GUIDELINES

INTRODUCTION

What is this book about?

This book is about the principles and practice of homeopathy. It is an introductory textbook which assumes no previous knowledge of homeopathy. It is intended to provide the reader with a good basic understanding of homeopathy and to allow him or her to begin to introduce homeopathy into their daily work within the primary health care team.

Homeopathy as a therapeutic option may be introduced to daily practice in two ways. Firstly, awareness of the possibilities which homeopathy can offer allows the practitioner to make relevant referrals to suitably qualified specialists. Secondly, knowledge of the basic principles of prescribing, in addition to knowledge of the main prescribing features of some remedies of use in commonly experienced clinical conditions, allows the practitioner to begin to add homeopathic prescribing to their personal range of clinical skills.

Who should read this book?

Any health care professional working within a primary care setting who wishes to be able to offer homeopathy as a therapeutic option to their patients.

This book is relevant to the work of general practitioners, (otherwise known as family practice physicians, primary care physicians, or family doctors), health visitors, community nurses and midwives, practice nurses, nurse practitioners and physician's assistants in particular, but will be of use to any other member of the primary care team who wishes to gain an understanding of homeopathy.

Why learn homeopathy?

Your patients are using it

Although homeopathy has been practised for over 200 years it has become particularly popular in recent years. This is partly due to the general public's increased interest in 'complementary medicine'.

The results of two surveys carried out by the Consumers' Association in the UK showed an increase in public use of complementary therapies from one in seven of their membership in 1985 to one in four by 1991.

An editorial in *Health Bulletin* by the Chief Medical Officer in Scotland in 1983 concluded that 'Alternative medicine is giving our patients something they value which we are failing to provide them with'.

Similar increases in public use of complementary therapies in general, and homeopathy in particular, are being reported through-out Europe and the USA.

The British Medical Association, in their 1993 publication, *Complementary Medicine. New Approaches to Good Practice*, concluded that:

> *One of the main reasons for the current upsurge of official interest in non-conventional medicine is the rapidly increasing number of patients who are seeking help from such practitioners. This has prompted the Council of Europe to state 'It is not possible to consider this phenomenon as a medical side-issue. It must reflect a genuine public need which is in urgent need of definition and analysis.*

This popularity means that you are increasingly likely to discover that your patients are using homeopathy or are going to ask you for a referral to a homeopathic specialist.

Your colleagues are using it.

Several studies have shown that large numbers of health care pro-fessionals either practise complementary therapies themselves or wish to see such therapies become more available to their patients.

In the UK, the Faculty of Homoeopathy is the statutory recognized body which oversees standards of training and the practice of homeo-pathy by doctors and other registered health care professionals. The Faculty has a membership of over 600 practising doctors in the UK.

Several studies of doctors' attitudes to complementary therapies have shown the majority of doctors to be sympathetic and, in fact, in one study (Anderson & Anderson. JRCGP 1987) 95% of doctors said they had discussed complementary therapies with patients in the previous year. Lothian Health, in Scotland, ran a pilot homeopathic clinic in 1994 and found that 40% of all Lothian family doctor practices made a referral to the clinic within the first 4 weeks of setting it up.

Surveys conducted by the Academic Departments of Glasgow Homeopathic Hospital have shown that 20% of all Scottish family doctors have attended at least one part of the postgraduate courses in homeopathy run in Glasgow. The Glasgow courses are, in fact, the most popular courses in postgraduate medical education, in any discipline, in the whole of the UK.

Is homeopathy 'complementary' or 'alternative'?

'Alternative medicine', 'complementary medicine', 'unorthodox medicine', 'non-conventional medicine' and even 'traditional medicine' are all terms used to try and classify homeopathy. The terms 'complementary' and 'alternative' , in particular, cause great confusion.

Homeopathy does not really require any more classification than its own self-explanatory name. However, the terms 'complementary' and 'alternative' seem to hint at different ways of using homeopathy, or even different views of the place of homeopathy in the rich menu of therapeutic options on offer to a 'sick' person.

The question is whether homeopathy is an entire system of medicine rivalling modern Western medicine or an adjuvant, to be used only alongside other therapies. As far as individual patients are concerned, the argument is specious. Modern Western medicine has shown enormous progress in the 20th century. In particular, great strides have been made in the management of acute disease. Doctors are much better at saving lives now. The greatest challenge to doctors, however, is still the area of 'cures'. Chronic diseases, in particular, still evade 'cure'. Homeopathy has claimed an ability to effect 'cures'. Can this claim be justified? We will examine the evidence later.

Once you have learned homeopathy and can begin to introduce it to your daily work, you will find that there are many circumstances where you choose a homeopathic option for a patient because you believe it is the best available option, i.e. the alternative options are inferior. There will be other clinical situations where you will choose to use a homeopathic option in association with other therapeutic interventions, i.e. using it in a truly 'complementary' manner. The therapist's duty is to find the most appropriate range of therapeutic options for any individual patient, not to be hidebound by dogma.

Why use homeopathy in your practice?

No effective allopathic alternative exists

There are many clinical conditions for which there are no effective allopathic treatments. On a daily basis we find ourselves unable to come up with a cure, or even a treatment, for both acute and chronic diseases. Later in the book we shall look at specific examples.

This will probably be the area of clinical practice where you first introduce homeopathy as an option.

The clinical situation makes an allopathic option unsafe

Pregnancy, breastfeeding, impaired renal or hepatic function often require that the allopathic option is chosen only with great care. Homeopathic remedies are completely safe in these areas. They can be used without risk of toxicity.

The side-effect profile of the allopathic option makes it unacceptable

Many allopathic drugs are toxic or have serious side-effects. Non-steroidal antiinflammatories are notorious for their damaging effects on the gastrointestinal tract. Homeopathic remedies have no such side-effects or toxicity.

Reduction in amount of chronic allopathic treatment

Many chronic conditions can be suppressed with allopathic drugs to enable an improved quality of life and even life expectancy. However, all allopathic drugs are toxic and as practitioners we are often attempting to find long-term drug regimes which involve the smallest amounts or shortest courses of these 'necessary' drugs. A good example of this is asthma, where steroids have shown enormous benefit but, due to their toxicity, it is important to use as little of them as possible whilst allowing the patient to receive the maximum benefit.

Homeopathic remedies can be used, in this situation, in a 'complementary' manner to minimize the need for the more toxic drugs.

Rewards of using homeopathy in your practice

The practice of homeopathy brings the practitioner an enormous number of rewards. Indeed, it is the personal satisfaction brought about by these rewards which 'hooks' practitioners into continuing their study of and practice of homeopathy for the rest of their lives! The rewards come in various forms.

Making a difference – patient satisfaction

Patients who have been helped by the homeopathic treatments you have given them tend to let you know. They may stop you in the street to tell you how much better they feel since you gave them the 'wee white tablets' or they may simply ask for a homeopathic treatment in the future. Either way, the patient feedback from those who have benefited from homeopathic treatment is impressive and tends to exceed that from patients who have felt an improvement from an allopathic treatment.

Making a difference – practitioner satisfaction

Most of us decided to enter this profession because we wanted to be involved in 'healing'. Most of us quickly discover that our daily practice does not involve us in much 'healing'. Therefore, when we do manage to make a difference – a difference which patients feel is of significance in their daily living – then we get in touch with the reasons we chose this profession in the first place.

Making sense of our daily work – the effect on consultation style

The process of understanding a patient and being able to work out the most suitable homeopathic remedies for them involves us in approaching the patient in a more 'holistic' way and in trying to understand their individuality as part of the diagnostic process. This results in us having to become better listeners and, in a traditional sense, become better at consulting – better at eliciting a relevant history, better at facilitating the patient's communication with you and better at responding to the patient.

Therefore, even before a homeopathic remedy is prescribed, the quality of your work has improved. This improvement brings a greater sense of reward and purpose to our work.

Making sense of our daily work – understanding aetiology

The homeopathic theory of the origins of 'illness' in an individual enables us to better understand the aetiology of the patient's condition. We ask ourselves the questions: Why is this person suffering from this 'illness' at this time? Where did this 'disturbance' of health come from?

Making sense of our daily work – understanding patterns of disease

The homeopathic understanding of the behaviour of 'illness' helps us to make sense of prognosis and to see the patterns of 'illness' in both families and communities. This also helps us to understand the relevance of our daily work.

Mental rewards – the joy of detective work

One of the challenges of medicine is to arrive at the diagnosis. In homeopathic terms this includes a full understanding of the individual who is suffering from the 'illness'. Eliciting the relevant 'clues' and 'insights' to be able to arrive at this understanding is highly rewarding.

Mental rewards – a sense of intellectual achievement

The study of homeopathy can become a life's work. There are over 2000 remedies available to the homeopathic practitioner. Learning the 'drug pictures' of these remedies and then recognizing these patterns in the 'illnesses' of our patients brings a great sense of intellectual achievement. In recognition of our learning, standard

HOMEOPATHY IN PRIMARY CARE

examinations are available. For example, in the UK, the Primary Health Care Certificate in Homoeopathy, accredited by the UK Faculty of Homoeopathy, can be gained by examination after a basic level of training. The US, at time of writing, is in the process of making available the same examination and the same certificate, accredited jointly by the UK Faculty of Homoeopathy and the American Board of Homeotherapeutics. For those medical practitioners who wish to practise homeopathy at a specialist level it is possible to gain 'Membership of the Faculty of Homoeopathy' by clinical examination.

Both these certificates bring a sense of intellectual achievement and mark this achievement within our peer group and within society at large.

WHAT IS HOMEOPATHY?

1

The basic principles

There are only two basic principles of homeopathy: treatment of 'like with like' and use of the minimum effective dose.

'Like cures like'

This is the essence of homeopathy.

This principle was discovered by Dr Samuel Hahnemann in the second half of the 18th century. Hahnemann was translating Cullen's Materia Medica from English into German when he came across a description of the action of Peruvian tree bark in the treatment of swamp fever. Hahnemann began to speculate about why this particular substance cured swamp fever. To investigate, he took some of the tree bark himself and discovered to his surprise that he developed the same pattern of symptoms as that of a person suffering from swamp fever. In other words, the medicine which produced the cure of an illness was capable of inducing the same symptoms of the illness when given to a healthy person. This phenomenon was then shown to be reproducible in a range of 'cures'.

Having discovered this natural phenomenon, he then went on, experimentally, to discover the 'pictures' of other drugs and treat patients with them. Homeopathy is still based on this discovery.

In each case of 'illness' the homeopathic practitioner has to know two things – the patient and the cure.

The 'picture' of the patient's illness is ascertained through a thorough examination of the patient by careful history taking, along with observation and physical examination of the patient. This enables the practitioner to make a clear diagnosis and also to be aware of the specific features of the 'illness' in this particular individual. The practitioner then attempts to work out which medicinal substance has a 'drug picture' which most closely resembles the 'picture' of the 'illness' in this patient.

An example commonly experienced in primary care is that of the preschool febrile child. A typical picture would be flushed cheeks, dry mouth, dilated pupils, agitation and, perhaps, even frightening hallucinations. A very similar pattern of symptoms could be induced in a healthy child by administering Belladonna (deadly nightshade). Vasodilation, dry mucous membranes, dilated pupils and delirium are all features of poisoning by the atropine-like substances found in Belladonna.

Homeopathic treatment of this child would consist, therefore, of giving a remedy prepared from Belladonna. Obviously, the dose should not be so high as to cause poisoning of the child. This leads to the second principle of homeopathic treatment – the use of the minimum effective dose.

The Minimum Effective Dose

The therapeutic agents used in homeopathy are called 'remedies'. Clearly, many medicinal substances are potentially extremely toxic. The active element in Peruvian tree bark turns out to be quinine (and swamp fever is now known to be malaria).

One of the problems with the treatment of swamp fever with Peruvian tree bark in Hahnemann's day was the toxicity of the original substance. In preparing useful remedies from the substances Hahnemann had examined, he attempted to find the minimum effective dose, i.e. the least amount of the medicine required to have the desired therapeutic effect. In the 18th century physicians prepared their own medicinal substances. Hahnemann prepared his remedies by producing a series of dilutions in alcohol. With each stage of dilution he vigorously shook the substance – a process known as 'succussion'.

When he used the remedies in practice he found, again to his surprise, that the more stages of dilution and succussion the substance had undergone, the greater its therapeutic effect on the patients. For this reason he called the process 'potentization' and the remedies were then known as 'potencies'.

Up to this point you will probably not have read anything you would consider to be controversial. So, why isn't homeopathy more widely accepted? The clue lies in the limits to which the process of serial dilutions and succussions is carried. The remedies used in practice have typically undergone 30 of these stages and in some cases they have undergone several thousand. This is where homeopathy begins to get controversial. If these remedies have been subjected to so many dilutions and succussions, then how can they be active? Surely there are no molecules of the original active substance left at such high dilutions?

We will look at these questions in detail later.

Key points

- The two basic principles of homeopathy are:
  1. treatment of 'like with like';
  2. use of the minimum effective dose.
- Homeopathic 'drugs' are known as 'remedies'.
- Homeopathic remedies are prepared using a process of multiple dilutions and 'succussions'. This process is known as 'potentization'.
- The greater the number of stages of potentization, the greater the therapeutic potential of the remedy.

HOW ARE REMEDIES PREPARED? 2

The homeopathic pharmacopœiae of America, Germany, Britain and France give detailed instruction on the preparation of remedies and set out standardized methods of dealing with the various types of raw materials used.

The raw materials

A common misconception is that homeopathic remedies are herbal remedies. It is true that about 70% of all homeopathic remedies are prepared from plants. However, the remaining 30% are prepared from other natural sources such as minerals, animals and from any substances which can induce disease. The plant remedies include some well-known plants such as deadly nightshade (Belladonna) and bitter cucumber (Colocynthis). Some of these plants contain toxins, but they are rendered completely harmless by the process of serial dilutions and successions. Interestingly, some of the plants are used by both herbalists and homeopathic practitioners to treat the same clinical conditions. For example, the homeopathic remedy Caulophyllum is used in the treatment of women in labour. The same plant is known to the Native Americans as squaw root and was traditionally chewed by squaws during labour. This overlap of prescribing indication between homeopathic remedies and herbal products is, perhaps, one of the reasons for the confusion which exists in the public understanding of these two therapies.

Mineral sources of homeopathic remedies are numerous and include substances which are relatively inert chemically, such as Silica, as well as toxic chemicals, such as Arsenic. Sources from the animal world provide some of the most interesting remedies. A good example of this is Lachesis, which is a remedy prepared from the venom of the bushmaster snake. The remedy is useful in certain forms of premenstrual syndrome, with some of its keynotes being 'feelings of constriction – especially around the neck' and 'sudden flashes of aggression'. The behaviour of the snake from which this venom is taken includes sudden, darting aggression and constriction of its prey.

Finally, any substances which cause ill health can be 'potentised', i.e. made into remedies. Examples of these include remedies prepared from allergens and given to patients as part of a programme of desensitization. Perhaps the best known of these are house dust mite and grass pollens.

Preparation of remedies

The first stage in the preparation of a remedy is to produce a 'mother tincture'. A mother tincture is a liquid form of the original substance dissolved in alcohol or water, depending on its solubility. There are three forms of mother tincture:

1. Essence – prepared from the juice expressed from plants and preserved in 90% alcohol;
2. Tincture – 60–90% alcohol used to extract the active constituents from powdered dried plants or from crushed animal material, e.g. bees;
3. Solution – soluble minerals dissolved in water or alcohol according to their solubility.

In the case of insoluble materials, such as minerals, the raw material is ground into lactose powder with a mortar and pestle for one hour. The resulting substance is known as an 'original trituration'.

Potentization

There are two elements to the process of potentization – serial dilution and succussion.

There are three 'scales' of potentization used in the world, with each scale referring to the amount of dilution at each stage. The two commonest are the 'decimal' and the 'centesimal' scales. In the decimal scale each stage of dilution is in the ratio of one part substance to nine parts diluent (ethyl alcohol). In the centesimal scale each stage of dilution is in the ratio of one part substance to 99 parts diluent. The third, less commonly used scale is the 'LM' scale, developed by Hahnemann using sugar granules, in which each stage is a 50 000th dilution.

There are two traditional methods of preparing the potencies. Hahnemann's method is known as the 'multiple vial method'. In this method, to prepare a 30c potency, 30 vials are taken and 99 parts of ethyl alcohol are added to each one. One part of the mother tincture is then added to the first vial which is then succussed (ten rapid downward motions of the vial). One part is then taken from the first vial and added to the second vial which is then succussed and then the process continues in sequence to the 30th vial. As this method is expensive (all the intervening potencies up to the 30th are discarded), the 'single vial method' was introduced by Korsakoff, who noted that when liquid is tipped out of a vial a little liquid is left behind. He measured the amount left behind and found that, on average, it was equivalent to one drop. In this method, the potency is tipped out of the vial and then 99 drops are added to the 'empty' vial to prepare the next potency. Although less expensive, this method is not as accurate as the multiple vial method. However, no studies have demonstrated any differences in efficacy between the two methods.

The final liquid potency is applied to a delivery agent, usually a tablet or powder of lactose. The powders are traditionally dispensed in tens and the tablets are sold by weight with 7 g and 25 g being standard sizes.

Potencies will be discussed later but a wide range are used, some of which undergo an astonishing number of dilutions in their preparation. For example, a 30c has undergone 30 stages of 1:99 dilution, giving a final dilution of 100^{30}. Dilutions undergoing 1000 or more stages are designated by the letter 'M'. A 1M is therefore the result of 1000 stages of 1:99 dilutions.

Obviously, once a solution has undergone such a high number of dilutions, it is extremely unlikely that even a single molecule of the original substance is left. This is probably the most controversial aspect of homeopathic practice. To the scientific mind, trained in molecular biology, this doesn't make sense. However, as scientists, our approach should not be to try to fit the evidence into our existing theories, but to examine the evidence and then produce some theories consistent with that evidence.

Key points

- Three common scales of potencies:
  1. Decimal (X or D);
  2. Centesimal (c), with 1000c represented as 1M;
  3. LM (1 in 50 000).
- Two main methods of preparation:
  1. Hahnemannian – multiple vial method;
  2. Korsakoff – single vial method.
- Starting solution known as mother tincture.
- Insoluble substances rendered soluble by trituration – grinding and mixing substance with lactose powder.

IS THERE A PHENOMENON HERE? 3

The concept of microdilutions having a biological effect challenges our current scientific understanding. The greatest stumbling block to mainstream acceptance of homeopathy by the scientific establishment is the claim that dilutions which, theoretically, are extremely unlikely to contain any molecules whatsoever can produce a biological effect. The reason this is a stumbling block is due entirely to the current dominance of the paradigm of molecular biology.

These issues are examined in more detail later in this chapter. However, as we begin to try to make sense of the use of these extremely high dilutions, the first question to ask ourselves is not 'How does this theory fit with other scientific theories?' but 'Is there a phenomenon here?'. Can we find any evidence to suggest that homeopathy actually does anything at all? Can we find any evidence to suggest that it actually works? There are two main areas to examine – clinical research and clinical experience.

Clinical research

For many years, critics of homeopathy have claimed that there is no evidence that homeopathy works. In fact, there is a substantial body of scientific evidence, with major research being published in main-stream medical scientific literature in the last 10 years.

Much work has been conducted in vitro with homeopathically prepared dilutions of substances. This work is of a highly technical nature. The interested reader should consult some of the following references.

Homeopathy – A Frontier in Medical Science, by Bellavite and Signorini contains an excellent survey of laboratory experiments.

The more accessible and more exciting work is the clinical trial data, published in the major medical journals.

In 1986 David and Morag Taylor Reilly, of the Glasgow Homoeopathic Hospital, and their co-workers published 'Is Homoeopathy a placebo response?' in *The Lancet*. Using a standard randomized, double-blind control trial with crossover, this group compared the effects of a homeopathic preparation of grass pollens (prepared to a 30c potency, i.e. beyond the probability of the preparation containing any grass pollen molecules) against the effects of a placebo. They demonstrated statistically significant superiority of the homeopathic preparation over the placebo. This remains a robust well-accepted study. The Taylor Reilly team went on to conduct further studies using the same model and published again in *The Lancet* in 1994. This paper, entitled 'Is evidence for homoeopathy reproducible?', repeated the demonstrated superiority of the homeopathic preparation over placebo in a traditional randomized, double-blind control trial – the accepted medical scientific 'gold standard'. This paper provoked the Editor of *The Lancet* to write an editorial entitled 'Reilly's challenge' which concluded that either homeopathy worked or the randomized control trial didn't. He felt both conclusions were alarming.

In 1991, Kleijnen, Knipschild and Riet published a major review of clinical trials in homeopathy in the *British Medical Journal*. This review found 108 papers with 'interpretable' results, 81 of which showed a 'positive' outcome for homeopathy. In fact, this group analysed the scientific merit of the papers and showed that the greater the scientific merit, the more likely the trial was to show a positive effect of the homeopathy. They concluded that 'The evidence presented in this review would probably be sufficient for establishing homeopathy as a regular treatment for certain conditions'.

Gibson et al (1980) showed that 82% of patients in their treatment group reported improvement (in terms of pain, stiffness and articular index), as opposed to 21% in the placebo group.

The study by Ferley et al (1989) examined Oscillococcinum (a French homeopathic preparation from duck liver and heart) in the treatment of flu-like illnesses and showed a statistically significantly greater effect in producing cures within 48 hours than the placebo group.

Fisher et al (1989) reported a study that involved a clinical diagnosis of 'fibromyalgia' using accepted criteria, then taking a homeopathic history to see which of these patients would benefit from homeopathic Rhus Toxicodendron, then randomizing this group to receive

HOMEOPATHY IN PRIMARY CARE

Rhus Toxicodendron or placebo. The homeopathically treated group, in this double-blind study, had a better response.

Dorfman et al (1987) showed a combination of homeopathic remedies taken daily through the ninth month of pregnancy, compared to placebo in a double-blind study, to be significantly effective in reducing both duration of labour and the incidence of cervical dystocia.

Brigo & Serpelloni (1991) reported on the homeopathic treatment of migraine. In this study with good methodology, 100 patients with migraine were seen by a homeopathic doctor who selected 60 of them as presenting a clear homeopathic picture. This group was then randomized to receive either the remedy or placebo in a double-blinded manner. Follow-up over a few months showed significant benefit of the homeopathy over placebo.

The study on acute childhood diarrhoea published by Jacobs et al (1994) was a landmark because it was accepted for publication by a mainstream American medical journal. Again, the standard randomized double-blind method was used to compare homeopathic treatment against placebo, with all the children receiving oral rehydration therapy. The homeopathically treated children experienced a significant reduction in duration and intensity of their diarrhoea compared to the control group.

For those readers interested in examining more of the published evidence, the review paper by Knipschild, published in the *British Medical Journal*, is an excellent starting point and contains many references.

Clinical Experience

Clinical experience is, of course, the foundation on which the subject of homeopathy is built. Hahnemann repeatedly emphasized the value of observation and experimentation over theorizing. The core of the materia medicae used today is the evidence from 'provings' and from clinical experience in the form of published, repeatedly observed, 'cured symptoms' from practitioners' case histories.

In more recent years, the evidence of clinical experience has become more accepted by the scientific community within the context of 'clinical audit' and 'outcome studies'. An example of this kind of data is the following, as yet unpublished work from the Glasgow Homoeopathic Hospital.

David Reilly and his colleagues at the Glasgow Homoeopathic Hospital have developed a simple outcome measure which is being used at the hospital and by a large network of UK GPs who are collecting data using a standardized form and sending it to the Data Collection Unit at the Hospital. Any reader who would like to participate in this work should contact The Data Collection Manager, Academic Departments, Glasgow Homoeopathic Hospital, 1000 Great Western Road, Glasgow G12 ONR, Scotland, UK.

The outcome score uses the patient's language and relates the changes, if any, to the effect on the daily lives of the patients. 0 represents 'No change or unsure'. The full scale is as follows:

+4 Cured or back to normal
+3 Significant improvement
+2 Moderate improvement, affecting daily living
+1 Slight improvement, no effect on daily living
 0 No change or unsure
−1 Slight deterioration, no effect on daily living
−2 Moderate deterioration, affecting daily living
−3 Significant deterioration
−4 Disastrous deterioration

This score has been used in an audit of 100 consecutive inpatients and 100 consecutive outpatients attending the Glasgow Homoeopathic Hospital. The analysis of these audits is shown in Table 3.1.

The score has also been used by a network of family doctors and other health care professionals attending the courses in homeopathy run by the Academic Departments of the Glasgow Homoeopathic Hospital. Early returns have shown over 65% of all homeopathic prescriptions audited are rated as +2 or greater, i.e. improvement of value in the daily lives of the patients treated.

Consistency of Theory

A third main strand in convincing practitioners that homeopathy does present a real phenomenon in healing which merits further consideration is the 'internal' consistency of the subject. Time and time again homeopathic practitioners witness the truth of the Materia Medica information. Every practitioner will have examples of patients who remark that symptoms which he or she had 'forgotten to mention' have improved after the treatment. When the practitioner consults the

Table 3.1 Audit of 100 sequential outpatients and inpatients at Glasgow Homoeopathic Hospital from July 1992, followed up after 1 year

Outpatients
60% improved in the presenting complaint
61% improved well-being
49% had sustained improvement of value in daily living
37% had a sustained reduction in conventional therapy

Inpatients
100% had already received conventional care
97% had already seen a consultant specialist in another speciality for this problem
67% had previously been admitted to other hospitals with this problem

3 months after treatment
58% had improvement in presenting complaint of value in daily living
67% had improvement in mood and well-being of value in daily living

Materia Medica picture of that remedy the 'unmentioned' symptom is often found to be one of the features of that remedy.

The association between the 'mental and general symptoms' (representing the patient's 'constitutional type') and 'local' or 'pathological' symptoms within distinct patterns as represented by the remedy pictures is also commonly seen.

So, it would seem that the evidence of our eyes and ears is that there is something happening here. The homeopathic method does produce results and does influence the health of the patients who receive homeopathic treatment. How can we make sense of this phenomenon?

Paradigm Shift

'A paradigm is a set of theoretical assumptions, experimental practices and modes of transmitting the contents of science' (Kuhn 1962).

The dominant paradigm is molecular biology. However, let us step behind this paradigm and consider the paradigm of information. (See also Graphic 1, p. 256.)

'Disease is ... essentially an information disorder' (Bellavite and Signorini). The human organism is a complex system and developments in systems analysis and the study of complex systems have helped us to see the human organism differently. 'The more complex a system, the more complex will be its communications strategy' (ibid.).

What is information? 'Information is the ability to establish order' (Harold). 'Information is the power to direct what is done' (Jacob). Our genetic code is, of course, our fundamental source of information. The interaction of this code with information received from the external and internal environments determines our well-being, our health, our very behaviour. The information our systems receive is sometimes molecular; examples include infectious agents such as bacteria and viruses and also 'designer molecules' in the form of 'drugs'. However, much of the information we receive is not molecular; examples include light, sound, heat, gravitational force and other forms of energy. Modern theories of physics are challenging the particulate and molecular bases of our understanding of reality.

Other forms of information may be quite complex. Language, for example, uses sound to convey information, but to try to reduce language to a science of sound waves leaves us with an inadequate understanding of it. This is seen at a further level of complexity when language is used in the form of literature. In 1995, the UK Poetry Society provided poets in residence in two general hospitals to conduct a study of the effects of poetry on health. Music is another example of the additional complexity of sound as an information source when the sound has a 'coherence' which conveys more than analysis of the sound waves will reveal.

The fact that such complex information can have real biological significance is understood by most people. Ailments which arise after emotionally traumatic events, such as the death of a loved one, are seen by doctors on a daily basis. 'Information' in this sense is only a part of communication. The 'meaning' we give to this 'information' is the result of an interaction between the information source and the recipient of the information.

An interesting analogy using these concepts is to think of the sick patient as being lost in a maze. Any therapeutic intervention is an attempt to enable the patient to find his or her way out of this maze, back to health. The interventions which are most effective are 'maps' of the maze. Using the correct 'map' allows the patient to find his or her way out. Homeopathic remedies are, in this way of thinking, simply 'maps'. Taking this idea a little further, an allopathic drug is probably more akin to a set of directions than a map. The drug 'says' take the first left, the second right and so on. It often fails to cure completely because the directions are incomplete and do not empower the patient to find another way out if the road is blocked due to unforeseen circumstances.

So we understand that information in many forms can have an effect on health. How is the information being conveyed in the homeopathic method? How much information is conveyed in the remedy and how much in the process of the therapeutic technique? These are very difficult questions and they highlight an expanse of scientific ignorance in the processes of disease and healing. How does any healing take place? What are the essential components? Why doesn't the same drug have the same therapeutic power in two individuals with the 'same' disease? These are the questions at the frontier of medical science. However, for the purposes of this study of homeopathy, suffice it to say that we no longer require a molecular understanding of disease and healing. The information paradigm can release us from that mental straitjacket.

The other major paradigm which is in the ascendancy is the holistic one. With increased understanding of the interconnectedness of molecules, cells, tissues and systems (neurological, endocrine, immunological), we are more likely now to consider disease within the context of the whole patient. This is not a new idea. In the 19th century, Osler said 'It is better to know the patient who has the disease, than the disease which has the patient' (Osler 1892). A leading article in the *British Medical Journal* in recent years had the title 'Irritable bowel? Irritable body? Irritable brain?' and considered the evidence for a whole-person disorder of which bowel 'irritability' was only a part. This article showed that we understand only certain aspects of a disease or disorder and treat only those.

Two further areas of study will challenge our understanding of the processes of disease and healing – the placebo phenomenon and the emerging science of psychoneuroimmunology (PNI).

A study in the *World Journal of Surgery* in 1983 reported a randomized controlled trial of two chemotherapy protocols in gastric cancer. The patients in the 'control' placebo group experienced side-effects of the 'placebo'. In fact, 34.6% experienced drug-related nausea, 21.5% drug-related vomiting and an astonishing 30.8% suffered hair loss.

One of the most famous and amazing stories about the power of the placebo was the story of Mr Wright who was suffering from a lymphatic tumour and who was admitted to hospital expecting to die. At this time a new chemotherapeutic agent – Krebiozen – was launched with great claims of its power. Mr Wright was given Krebiozen and had a dramatic response, with his tumour size shrinking enormously, and he was discharged from the hospital 10 days after his treatment. All went well until 2 months later when some adverse reports were published suggesting that trial data had shown that Krebiozen was ineffective. Mr Wright went into relapse and was readmitted.

At this point his doctors decided to try an experiment. They told him that a super-refined, double-strength Krebiozen had been made and they were getting some for him, but that it would take a few days. After a few days they injected him with sterile water, having told him this was the new wonder drug. He again underwent amazing improvement, was discharged and remained well until the American Medical Association announced that extensive trials had shown Krebiozen to be 'worthless'. Within a few days Mr Wright died.

In dentistry, it has been shown that 40% of patients with postextraction dental pain receive pain relief from placebo agents. A study in *Nature* in 1983 showed that in a group of these patients given naloxone, 50% started to complain of pain again, suggesting that the placebo pain relief must involve the production of natural opiates – the endorphins.

These stories show the power of the placebo response. They also tend to disguise the serious questions behind this phenomenon and in the medical profession the concept of the placebo has become confused with the concept of 'unreal' or 'pretend' treatment. There is nothing 'unreal' or 'pretend' about the power of this phenomenon to affect health. Indeed, we are probably witnessing the same human phenomenon when we see the effects of death of a spouse and the studies of the phenomenon of 'significant dates', where both 'deadlines' and 'lifelines' have been demonstrated. A 'deadline' is shown in the fact that many people die at the same age at which their parents die. A 'lifeline' is shown in the fact that three US presidents have died on 4th July.

The 'placebo effect' is probably a part of every therapeutic intervention. It can be demonstrated just as powerfully in the scenario of serious organic pathology, e.g. cancer, as in the scenario of psychosomatic disease. It is therefore not a diagnostic tool. Witnessing a healing response to a 'sham' therapeutic intervention does not help establish a diagnosis. In fact, it raises the question of 'What is a sham therapeutic intervention?'. The ubiquitous nature of the placebo response in therapeutic interventions has led David Reilly and others to propose changing the term 'placebo response' to 'self-healing response'.

Perhaps some light will be shed on this phenomenon by the emerging science of psychoneuroimmunology.

Key points

- There are many published reports of randomized controlled clinical trials demonstrating the effectiveness of homeopathy over placebo.
- There is a vast body of clinical evidence supporting homeopathy
- Molecules are not an essential part of the healing process.
- The field of psychoneuroimmunology is providing new insights into the essentially holistic, integrated nature of the human being – our disease processes and our healing processes.

Key references

Reilly D, et al 1994 Is evidence for homoeopathy reproducible? Lancet 344:1601

Kleijnen J, Knipschild P, 1991 Clinical trials of homoeopathy. British Medical Journal 302: 316

Jacobs J, et al 1994 Treatment of acute childhood diarrhoea with homoeopathic medicine: a randomized clinical trial in Nicaragua. Paediatrics 93:719

SINGLE REMEDY, SINGLE DOSE 4

There are many schools of homeopathy. As with many areas of study, whether in art or science, charismatic and powerful individuals acquire a following of students who, together, promulgate the 'great teacher's wisdom'. Overall, the classification of these schools developed and used by the French, is one of the most useful.

The Uniciste school teaches that each homeopathic prescription will be for a single homeopathic remedy given as a single dose. The practitioner will then arrange a follow-up visit at an appropriate interval and will make no further prescription until he or she has assessed the effect of the initial dose.

This was the original teaching of Samuel Hahnemann and this pattern of prescribing is often referred to as 'classical' homeopathy. It is the dominant school in most Western countries.

At the other end of the scale is the Complexiste school. This is so-called because the practitioners prescribe 'complexes' of homeopathic remedies. A complex of remedies contains several remedies in each 'pill'. The remedies are usually chosen with the patient's clinical diagnosis in mind and are likely to be the 'top 3' or 'top 10' most frequently indicated remedies for this clinical condition. An example of this is a travel sickness pill containing three common remedies for the treatment of travel sickness. The proponents of this school do not 'individualize' their prescriptions. The prescribing is led entirely by the diagnosis. This is obviously much easier and quicker than 'single dose, single remedy'. Most of the complex remedies available are for the treatment of acute conditions such as travel sickness, colds, sinusitis, dysmenorrhoea, etc. The remedies are taken as often as required and for as long as required.

The greatest criticisms of this technique are firstly a failure to individualize the prescription – the remedy prescribed is not chosen on the basis of the individual patient's reaction patterns – and secondly the difficulty in deciding what has helped and how to make the second prescription.

If the patient returns cured, then well and good. However, if the patient comes back and says that one of the major complaints is considerably better but two of the other complaints are worse and overall he or she feels no better, how does the practitioner know what components of the complex have helped?

Many of the complex remedies are marketed by homeopathic drug companies using trade names which clearly indicate the intended use. This means that they are easily understood by the public and are often purchased as 'over the counter' drugs without the guidance of a homeopathic prescriber.

In between these two schools is the Pluraciste school.

Here, the practitioner will determine that he or she wishes to prescribe a number of remedies for a single patient, on the basis of different aspects of the case history or of different prescribing strategies. The prescription issued will be for single remedies given in a staged manner. For example, the patient may be asked to take one dose of remedy A today, followed by one dose of remedy B twice daily for a week, followed by one dose of remedy C to be taken in 4 weeks time. The prescriber must have a clear idea of what he or she hopes to achieve with each of the remedies prescribed and will assess the responses to the various remedies on that basis at the follow-up visit. This school is most formally recognized in France, but much modern homeopathic prescribing is of this nature.

My own training is in the 'one remedy, one dose' school of prescribing and, whilst I have experimented with the other two systems, I remain most comfortable with that method, as it is based on individualization of the prescription and is the clearest method when trying to assess the response to the prescription.

Potency

Two of the words used most commonly in homeopathy have very therapeutic connotations – 'remedy' and 'potency'.

Homeopathic medicinal compounds are not generally referred to as 'drugs'. Instead, the commonly employed term is 'remedy'. This is very appropriate. By and large, drugs do not work with the human healing response. Rather, they suppress activity (witness the large number of drugs whose effects are 'anti-' something) or they replace a perceived 'deficiency', e.g. thyroxine, insulin, etc. Remedies on the other hand, are presumed to work by stimulating the human healing system. They are not thought to be suppressive.

The word 'potency' has the connotation of power. The nearest analogy would be 'strength'. 'Potency' is, in many ways, the homeopathic equivalent of 'dosage'. As we saw earlier, the preparation of remedies involves a series of dilutions and succussions. The stage of succussion between each stage of dilution is thought to be crucial. It is this stage which energizes, 'dynamizes' or 'potentizes' the preparation and which distinguishes the remedy from mere dilutions.

Each stage of preparation therefore yields a more powerful therapeutic tool, not a weaker one. This might lead the student to think that he or she should always choose the very highest potency available when making a prescription in order to achieve the maximum therapeutic potential. Sadly, life is never so simple! Clinical experience over the last couple of hundred years has shown that certain potencies are more effective in certain situations. This evidence, by the way, is purely a series of clinical observations handed down from teacher to student. There has not been any good research into this area of homeopathic practice, to date, and the student will encounter a bewildering range of beliefs and habits in relation to potency selection.

It should always be remembered that the most important step in prescribing is choosing the remedy. The selection of potency is a very secondary and frequently much more arbitrary step. As described earlier, two scales of potency are most commonly used – the decimal scale and the centesimal scale. In most countries, any potency below a 30c is referred to as a 'low potency', 30c is 'mid potency' and any potency greater than 30c is a 'high potency'. In France, there is a difference caused mainly by legislation which forbids the sale of remedies with a potency greater than 30c. This has led the French to develop and prescribe many more potencies below 30c and to refer to 30c as a 'high potency'.

The student's first homeopathic prescriptions can safely be 30c; as this is 'mid potency' it will be, in most cases, a reasonable opening prescription. However, there are widely held rules of potency selection. I stress that these rules are not rigid as they are the result of experience and habit.

Potency selection relates to a number of axes:

- acute/chronic – the more acute, the lower the potency;

- physical/emotional – the more physical the problem, the lower the potency;
- the 'vitality' of the patient – the lower the 'vitality', the lower the potency;
- the prescriber's fear of an aggravation – the greater the fear, the lower the potency;
- the confidence of the prescriber – the lower the confidence, the lower the potency.

Direction of cure

This began as an observation and, over time, has been given the status of a 'law', named after the doctor who first described it – Hering's Law. In fact, it is not a 'law' but simply an observation which many practitioners have seen for themselves. It tends to be used by practitioners in the analysis of the progress of chronic disease states. If change is occurring within the parameters of Hering's Law, the prescriber is likely to be happy to watch and to wait, without further prescription. Progress within the parameters is taken as evidence of remedy activity.

The direction of cure has four axes:

1. From most important organs to less important ones.
2. From inside, out.
   These first two can be seen in action where a patient with allergic asthma and eczema will experience an improvement in lung symptoms before an improvement in skin symptoms.
3. From top to bottom.
   Generalized skin eruptions will tend to improve on the head and face, then the trunk and then the limbs.
4. Disappearance of symptoms in reverse chronological order of their appearance.

That is, the most recent symptoms get better before the more long-standing ones. This process may also see the reappearance of 'old' symptoms which had been overtaken by more recent ones.

Changes in the patient's condition which follow a direction exactly contrary to this law are taken as evidence of the action of a 'wrong' remedy and the prescriber will try to antidote the current remedy and prescribe a more suitable one.

Key points

- Three schools of homeopathy – single remedy/single dose; multiple remedies in one pill; multiple remedies staged over time.

- Potency selection relates to a number of axes:
  1. acute/chronic;
  2. physical/emotional;
  3. the 'vitality' of the patient;
  4. the prescriber's fear of an aggravation;
  5. the confidence of the prescriber.

- The direction of cure has four axes:
  1. from most important organs to less important ones;
  2. from inside to ouside;
  3. from top to bottom;
  4. disappearance of symptoms in reverse chronological order of their appearance.

Taking a homeopathic history

5

The guidance and issues outlined in this chapter relate to the taking of a full homeopathic history. However, as in the rest of medicine, history taking is a seamless continuum from brief to comprehensive, with the chosen point on the continuum being determined by clinical appropriateness. The principles of history taking therefore apply throughout this range.

Firstly, however, what is a 'homeopathic consultation'? Any consultation is potentially homeopathic but it becomes so when the practitioner chooses to open up the possibility of a homeopathic treatment for the patient. Why might the practitioner choose to do this?

When a practitioner has recently been focusing on a particular therapeutic technique, he or she will see many opportunities to apply this technique. This arises from the practitioner's enthusiasm for the subject, mixed with their belief in their own skill in this area. One of the benefits of continuing education from one of the organizations offering homeopathic teaching is that your enthusiasm will receive regular boosts and this will lead to your thinking about the possibility of homeopathic treatment with more of your patients.

Colleague referral

Once it becomes known that you have developed an interest and some skill in homeopathy, your colleagues will begin to refer some of their patients to you. Beware! This may be flattering, but there is a well-established tendency of colleagues to refer to you their 'heart sink' patients, their most difficult cases. Remember that it takes many years of study and experience to become an expert. Don't bite off more than you can chew. Even after many years of developing your homeopathic skills it is unlikely that you will be able to cure all the patients that everyone else has failed with. In your early days of homeopathic practice perhaps it is best to remember the advice we give to children – 'Just say no to strangers'.

Patient request

Word of your interest in homeopathy will spread remarkably quickly. Increasingly you will be asked by patients for a homeopathic treatment option. 'I've come to you because you do homeopathy.' Such an opening gambit in a consultation does, of course, open the possibility of a homeopathic consultation. However, it does not guarantee it. As the therapist you may still decide that a homeopathic option is not in the patient's best interests or that the problem is of such duration and complexity that it is beyond your current skill level and you will refer the patient to a homeopathic specialist.

Well-established indication

Sometimes the patient's presenting symptoms constitute what is referred to as a 'well-established indication', in other words, a clinical situation which has repeatedly shown itself to be amenable to a particular homeopathic treatment. The use of Arnica in the treatment of a patient with bruises sustained during a fall is a good example.

Strange, rare or peculiar symptom

This provokes a homeopathic approach in a similar way to the above example of a 'well-established indication'. Often, however, a 'strange, rare or peculiar' symptom fails to lead the practitioner to a homeopathic prescription because, despite the unusual and striking nature of the symptom, the practitioner is unable to discover any remedy pictures which include this symptom.

The two goals of a homeopathic consultation

Firstly, to understand the patient and his or her illness. Secondly, to

HOMEOPATHY IN PRIMARY CARE

find an appropriate remedy. Too often a practitioner fails because they have lost the patient whilst looking for the remedy.

'The aims of case-taking are initially the same as in modern medicine generally. A diagnosis is to be made where possible. The prognosis is determined and assessed. A treatment plan is drawn up' (Koelher 1986, pp. 68–85). So again, the principle of maintaining your usual professional approach is important. Diagnosis and prognosis precede treatment. This order of priority has been around since ancient times. In *The Yellow Emperor's Classic of Medicine* (200–300 years BC), there is a description of the five Failings of Physicians:

1. failing in diagnosis;
2. failing in treatment, when physician neglects the patient's emotional experiences;
3. failing in deductive reasoning, without careful observation and history;
4. failing in counselling, lacking compassion and sincerity;
5. failing when simply inept and careless when administering medical care.

Note that the first four 'failings' relate to understanding the patient and his or her illness. The fifth is the only one which relates to the application of the therapy.

Let us consider that diagnosis and prognosis are therefore about understanding the patient. How can we do this effectively?

There are certain prerequisites or preconditions for good history taking, including both the physical environment and the practitioner's mental attitude. Vithoulkas (1986) states 'The environment should be quiet, with harmonious, simple, esthetic decor' (pp. 169–189). Koehler (1986) gives the following preconditions for good history taking: 'Calmness, time, patience, unbiased attitude, careful attention'.

Both of these authors are offering counsels of perfection. Most practitioners working in a primary care environment will find it difficult to meet these preconditions but it is worthwhile taking some time to consider these values in your daily task.

Take a sheet of paper and divide it into two columns. In the left-hand column write a list of aspects of your ideal internal and external environment in terms of encouraging good consultations with your patients. In the right-hand column, write a list of the actual internal and external environmental factors in which you work. Take a look at the differences. Don't get too depressed! Which of your ideal qualities seem achievable and how can you make some changes this week to move towards some of these ideals?

When taking the history, it is important to let the patient do most of the talking. Your first job is to record as faithfully as possible what the patient says. This is not an easy discipline, but it is an important one. The more you record your own words, rather than the patient's, the more you are likely to be making assumptions about what the patient is experiencing. This is a very great trap, both in orthodox medicine and in homeopathy. How many times have you heard a case history presented which is full of medical terminology which the patient neither used nor would understand? You will find that many homeo-pathic prescribers present case histories full of words and terms from the Repertory – words which the patient probably did not use.

Try to put yourself in the patient's shoes during the consultation. What exactly was the patient experiencing? Ask yourself if the picture you have of the patient is clear. One way to make a history clearer and to make sure you are getting the best understanding of the patient is to ask the patient for examples. For instance, if the patient says they are very irritable, ask them to describe the last time they felt irritable. When did it happen? What was happening? Who was there? How did that irritability feel? How was it expressed?

The elements of a full homeopathic history

There are three main 'sections' of a homeopathic history:

1. the conventional medical history;
2. the physiology of the patient;
3. the mental state.

We will examine these in detail one by one.

Conventional medical history

The conventional medical history has certain clearly defined areas of enquiry, starting with the presenting complaint. The important goals of this area are to record as much of the patient's story as possible and to encourage the patient to 'fill out' the detail of the symptoms, in order to obtain what the homeopathic prescriber calls 'complete symptoms'.

A complete symptom has four essential elements:

1. aetiology;
2. localization;
3. sensation;
4. modality.

Let us look at each of these in turn.

Aetiology. How did this symptom begin? Did it have a clear beginning and was that beginning provoked by any obvious event? Some examples of clear aetiology are injuries, bereavement and other equally traumatic events. The Repertory has a whole section in the 'Mind' chapter under 'Ailments from' which can give you some idea of what constitutes an aetiological factor.

Localization. A big word which just means 'Where is it?'. Where exactly is this sensation felt?

Sensation. What exactly is this sensation? Patients often have great difficulty describing a sensation. 'What is this pain like?' 'It's just sore.' 'But what kind of pain is it?' 'A sore pain.' Such a conversation can be very frustrating.

Tell the patient you want to understand what this pain feels like. Is it like having a knife stuck into you or does it feel more like having your inside tied in a knot? Beware, however, of giving such detailed examples as the patient might just opt for the first suggestion you give. Try to encourage the patient to express themselves in their own words first. If you have to give examples, then give two or three at least. Never slip into the bad practice of saying 'Is it a burning pain? No? Then is it a hammering pain?' and so on. Sooner or later, if you pursue this route, the patient is going to feel forced into agreeing with one of your answers. The answer will then be essentially your answer, not the patient's.

Modality

What modifies the sensation? What makes it feel worse (aggravates)? What makes it feel better (ameliorates)?

Following completion of the presenting complaint, the practitioner should then proceed to record the following:

- past medical history;
- family history;
- drug history;
- social history;
- Allergies
- systematic enquiry (a gathering of symptoms from the other body systems not already mentioned).

All of the above are standard to a medical history. The homeopathic equivalent is no different.

From this point on the history becomes somewhat different from the typical medical history. The differences are largely determined by the holistic nature of the homeopathic approach. As you will recall, the homeopathic prescriptions are individualized to the patient and it is not possible to make such a prescription without individualizing the history. We want to understand this person fully, not just their presenting problem. The symptoms noted during the detailed recording of the patient's presenting complaint are, largely, what homeopathic practitioners refer to as 'local symptoms', which tend to refer to only one part of the body, not to the whole body. Largely, these are pathological symptoms – the symptoms produced because of local pathology.

Physiology

The next major section is a consideration of the patient's physiology. These symptoms tend to be known as 'generals' and relate to the whole patient, not just to part of the patient.

Appetite. Is it increased or decreased? Is it variable? Is there an insatiable appetite? Is there easy satiety (does the patient quickly feel full when eating a meal)? There is more to appetite than simply absence or increase. A look at the symptoms listed under 'appetite' in the 'Stomach' chapter of the Repertory will give an idea of the potential scope.

Food. We are familiar with the phenomenon of cravings during pregnancy but the development of both food aversions and cravings is common outwith pregnancy. The patient should be asked if they have developed any craving or any aversions since they became unwell. The symptoms given spontaneously and with greatest intensity are, of course, the most valuable. Pay particular attention to any facial grimaces which accompany the expression of these symptoms, as these indicate a greater importance of the symptom. Also ask about food aggravations. Are there any foods which make any of the patient's symptoms worse?

The response to certain foods is frequently valuable. After the patient has spontaneously expressed the cravings, aversions and aggravations, he or she may be asked about some of these specifically. Salt, sweets, fat and dairy products are the main foods in this category. Obviously, great care should be taken over the eliciting of these responses. Patients will often tell you they dislike or avoid fat or sweets or salt because they know of the well-publicized healthy diet advice made much of by the medical profession and the media. When a patient says they never eat fat, they should be asked if, all the same, they do actually like the taste of it.

Thirst. Is it increased or decreased? Is there a surprising absence of thirst? What is the pattern of the thirst? Does the patient like small sips frequently or large quantities infrequently? What does the patient prefer to take to slake the thirst? Cold drinks or hot?

Sleep and dreams. Has the pattern of sleep changed? If so, in what way? In what position does the patient prefer to sleep? Has this changed since the illness began?

Can the patient recall his or her dreams? Are they disturbing? Are there any recurrent dreams or recurrent themes?

Temperature. We all have a preference for a particular atmospheric temperature. Some like it hot, others prefer the cool and yet others cannot bear the extremes of either temperature. What is the patient's preference in terms of atmospheric temperature? Has this changed since the patient became unwell?

This particular modality is often of great importance to the homeo-pathic practitioner but it only carries weight if it is a strong reaction. Some prescribers emphasize this by asking if this means the patient is a 'furnace' or an 'ice-man'.

Linked to temperature is the issue of perspiration. Is the perspira-tion profuse or scanty? Is it only on certain parts of the body? Is it offensive?

Weather. What are the effects of weather on the patient? This should be considered in terms of both 'locals' and 'generals'. This is a phenomenon which we all recognize but which has been largely disregarded by the medical profession. We all know patients who complain of painful muscles or joints in damp weather or headaches from exposure to the sun, but we tend to dismiss this information. In a homeopathic history such symptoms can be very useful. The commonest weather modalities relate to dampness, thunderstorms, sun and wind. Recently reported phenomena include the huge increase in admissions to UK hospitals due to acute exacerbations of asthma during thunderstorms in the summer of 1995.

One further atmospheric modality often reveals symptoms of interest – sea air. The patient should be specifically asked if they feel either better or worse by the sea.

Time. There are probably time modalities to most symptoms. Here the practitioner is not just interested in the time modalities of specific symptoms, but of the whole patient.

Time should be considered in its various different orders – annual, seasonal, monthly, weekly and daily. Many patients will tell you there is a time in every day when they feel at their most weak or their most ill. Such times should be noted. Many remedies have distinct time modalities. Monthly time modalities in women may, of course, be menstrual rather than monthly and the menstrual history should be carefully taken in its own right. A useful question to elicit menstrual modalities is 'Do you know your period is coming?'. If the answer is 'Yes', then follow up by enquiring how the patient knows her period is coming.

The mental state

This is a similar examination to that done in a standard psychiatric history, but not strictly the same.

This can be a difficult area to explore, but it is often of key importance, particularly in the management of chronic disease and in the individualization of the treatment. It is usually best left to last, allowing the patient to become comfortable with you and to have built up a certain degree of trust. However, this is not a hard and fast rule and as you become more experienced you will be able to introduce greater complexity to the structure of the consultation. At the outset, however, a clear, if relatively inflexible structure is more likely to yield results than an unclear, yet flexible one.

Two questions can be asked at the outset of this section. Both are 'difficult' questions but their answers can be very revealing.

1. How would you describe yourself?
2. How would others describe you?

List the responses, one feature per line, interspersing each of the responses with silence until the patient runs out of things to say. At this point go back down the list feature by feature, expanding them one by one, encouraging the patient to explain what they mean by each of them.

Once this area of enquiry is complete, you can then move into a more structured enquiry of mental symptoms. This can take the form of three main areas.

Cognitive function. Consisting of concentration, memory, the making of mistakes (oral or written) and delusions of thought. Delusions in this context cover not only psychotic symptoms but also strange or disordered beliefs, e.g. someone believing they are two people.

Emotional Symptoms. Anxieties (Are you a worrier? What things do you worry about?). Fears and phobias. Sadness, depression and apathy (emotional negativity and flatness). Lack of self-confidence. Irritability and anger, with particular attention being paid to the manner of the expression of anger and irritability. Sensitivity and tearfulness.

This leads to the final area which is the mental and emotional symptoms which appear in relationships. This includes the Five Cs: company, consolation, confrontation, contradiction and criticism. Let us examine these in more detail.

Company. How does the patient feel about company? Do they prefer to be with others when they don't feel well or do they prefer to be on their own? How do they respond to company?

Consolation. Distinct from the issue of company, how does the patient respond to consolation? Does it help or hinder them?

Confrontation. How does the patient respond to confrontation? Can they handle it? Can they produce it when it is required?

Contradiction. How does the patient respond to and deal with contradiction?

Criticism. How does the patient handle criticism? Does it stay with them for a long time afterwards? Do they harbour grudges?

Jealousy. The patient should be asked if they feel jealousy and, if they do, in what situations and how do they handle it?

Finally, there should be some exploration of the patient's sexual function. This is always a delicate issue and should be explored sensitively and appropriately.

Recording the history

The issues around where to record the patient's history will be discussed later but it is important to consider the technique of writing the history down in a manner which will facilitate decisions about treatment and interpretation of responses to the prescribed remedies.

One symptom per line

Due to the pressures of both time and space, primary care records are often extremely abbreviated and condensed. Giving each symptom a line to itself can seem quite an alien practice. However, there are many advantages, the greatest being that it allows the patient's words to be recorded verbatim and then each symptom is revisited and expanded as far as possible. This allows the patient the opportunity to speak freely without interruption yet the practitioner can go back and gain a fuller understanding of what has been said. The other main advantage is the simpler highlighting of significant symptoms for the purposes of case analysis and prescribing.

Underlining

A convention has arisen of underlining symptoms with one, two or three lines, depending on the weighting the practitioner wishes to give the symptom. Many prescribers have evolved their own personal definitions of the levels of underlining. If you create your own, do your best to use the underlining in a consistent manner. One scheme proposed by George Vithoulkas relates the underlining to the three qualities of clarity, intensity and spontaneity. The more of these qualities a symptom possesses, the more underlines it receives.

Margins

Clear wide margins down the side of each page can serve a number of functions. The space in the margins can be used to jot down objective observations made by the prescriber as the patient speaks.

HOMEOPATHY IN PRIMARY CARE

It can be used to write down possible remedies which come to the practitioner's mind in relation to the symptoms being expressed. It can be used to mark with an asterisk selected symptoms which have been used by the practitioner in drawing up a prescribing strategy. It can also be used to write down the page number from the Repertory of selected rubrics relevant to specific symptoms (see Chapter 6).

It is good practice to record two further items somewhere clearly in the case history. Firstly, reasons for prescribing remedy X. Make a note of the prescribing strategy you have chosen. This may take the form of references to rubrics in a repertory or prescribing indications from a materia medica. Secondly, have some standardized way of recording outcome so that you can easily see which remedies have been prescribed and what the response has been to each of them.

Some practitioners use custom-made recording sheets whilst taking the history. These have the advantage of helping the new practitioner to remember to ask all the relevant questions, but most practitioners find them too restrictive once they become a bit more adept at taking the history. Figure 5.1 is an example of such a sheet, which you may wish to photocopy and use in your records.

At their most extreme, such recording sheets can become so comprehensive that they can function as questionnaires to be completed by the patient before meeting the practitioner.

Key points

- The two goals of a homeopathic consultation are firstly to understand the patient and his or her illness and secondly, to find an appropriate remedy.

- A complete symptom has four essential elements:
  1. aetiology
  2. localization
  3. sensation
  4. modality.

- Underlining – the three qualities of clarity, intensity and spontaneity.

Case record sheet			Date:	
Name		D.O.B.		
Address		Identifier		
		Sex	m/f	
Tel		Occupation		

Complaint:

History of present illness:

Past medical history:

Family history:

Drug history (other treatments):

Social history:

Figure 5.1   An example of a case record sheet.

Local symptoms [systematic enquiry] (checklist below):

Head		Stomach	
Eye		Abdomen	
Ear		Bowels	
Nose		Urinary	
Throat		Genitalia	
Face		Back	
Mouth		Extremities	
Respiratory		Skin	

General symptoms (physiology):

Effects of:
  Heat
  Cold
  Weather

Perspiration

Appetite

Food:
  Desires
  Aversions
  Aggravations

Thirst

Sleep

Dreams

Menstrual cycle

Figure 5.1 (Continued.)

Mental symptoms :

Treatment:

Reasons for choice of treatment:

Follow-up:

Figure 5.1 (Continued.)

HOMEOPATHY IN PRIMARY CARE

Making Sense of it All 6

Analysing the information

Having taken a full history, you will find yourself facing a lot of writing. You now probably know a lot more about the patient than any other practitioner. Many patients at this point will tell you no-one has ever listened to them so attentively before and they may already be beginning to feel better. There is no doubt that such genuine interest on the part of the practitioner, coupled with an accepting, non-judgemental attitude, is therapeutically beneficial. The well-conducted consultation is a key ingredient in the success of the homeopathic process.

The next step consists of trying to understand what all this information means. What is the patient really suffering from? Exactly what is 'wrong' with this patient and how did it all come about? There are some well-established methodologies which will help you to decipher it.

To begin with, be clear that what you are trying to do first of all is understand the patient. Your second goal is to decide whether or not you consider it appropriate to prescribe a homeopathic remedy and your third goal is to work out which remedy you wish to prescribe.

Firstly, then, you need to be clear about the diagnosis. What is the clinical diagnosis? If you don't know, are there any examinations or investigations which would make it clearer for you?

Secondly, what is the prognosis? What is the natural history of this disease? To what extent do you consider the patient's symptoms to be reversible? Obviously, no known therapy can straighten severely physically deformed rheumatoid joints, but you might expect to reduce joint inflammation and thereby reduce pain and stiffness. In other words, in considering prognosis, work within the context of treatment goals. What is achievable? What do you hope to be able to offer the patient? (See also Graphic 3, p. 258.)

Let us now consider the questions of what is really wrong with this patient and how this came about. What symptoms are important to the patient? It is useful to record clearly which symptoms upset the patient to the greatest extent. Which symptoms are having the biggest impact on the patient's daily life?

Where is the level of disturbance? This is a concept which may be unfamiliar to you but it is a very useful one in all clinical situations. Is the disturbance peripheral, central or mental? A peripheral disturbance is a disturbance or a pathology mainly focused on a well-localized area, with little central or mental disturbance. Sports injuries are typically of this type. A damaged tendon or muscle is not an indication that the patient is generally ill. These symptoms are referred to as locals homeopathically.

A central disturbance involves the patient's physiology and therefore produces what are referred to as 'general' symptoms homeopathically. The early stage of an acute infectious disease is a good example of this type of disturbance. In such a situation the patient may be experiencing a fever, sweats, thirst, weakness and restlessness. The main focus is the physiology of the patient, although in most of these situations there will be some mental disturbance, such as irritability or mental dullness. The 'centre of gravity' of the case is, however, in the physiology, not in the mind.

The third and deepest level is the mental. Again, there may well be both 'general' and 'local' symptoms, but the focus is the mind. Acute anticipatory anxiety or acute grief are examples of this type.

How did these symptoms come about? When and where did they begin? What else was happening in life around this time? Had there been any significant changes or upsets in your life that year? Get as clear an idea of the aetiology as you can. It will help you to both make sense of the patient's complaint and choose a remedy.

Finally, ask yourself which symptoms you hope to ameliorate. What are you trying to treat?

At this point you should have a clear understanding of the patient and his or her illness. You are ready to decide whether or not you wish to treat this patient with a homeopathic remedy. Given that you do decide to prescribe a remedy, how do you decide which particular remedy to prescribe, which potency to choose and how frequently to give the remedy? There are two stages to this process. The first stage is to examine the symptoms you have recorded. The second stage is to determine a prescribing strategy.

First, let us look at the quality of the symptoms. Those which have

HOMEOPATHY IN PRIMARY CARE

the greatest importance are the 'strange, rare, peculiar' symptoms. Many beginners make the mistake of believing these to be the oddest, most bizarre symptoms (and many of these symptoms may be bizarre). However, the definition of 'strange, rare, peculiar' is broader than that in that the practitioner is looking for any symptom which is 'peculiar' to this patient. In other words, symptoms which one would expect from this pathology do not rank so highly. Most people with migraine get head pain but the rubric 'pain' in the Repertory chapter 'head' is too big to help you distinguish which remedy to use. A symptom which is less typical of those commonly reported by patients with migraine may be more indicative of this unique individual person. For example, if the patient with migraine says that the really frightening thing about his headache is that he goes completely blind with it but then, as the headache gets worse, the vision returns, then that is an unusual and potentially distinctive symptom which rates a higher significance in case analysis.

Another important quality marker of a symptom is the extent to which the symptom is volunteered spontaneously and said with emphasis. Both these features enhance the significance of the symptom.

A third quality marker is the 'completeness' of the symptom. Remember that a complete symptom has four aspects:

1. aetiology
2. sensation
3. localization
4. modality.

The final quality marker in determining symptoms of significance is deterioration. Any long-standing or new symptoms which are deteriorating have a strong potential to be significant.

Having examined the quality of the recorded symptoms we are now ready to assess the potential prescribing strategies. Over the years of homeopathic practice it has become apparent to practitioners that all symptoms, even if of equal quality, do not have equal significance in finding the most useful remedy. This has led to the evolution of the concept of a hierarchy of symptoms. The hierarchy is as follows (ranked with most important first):

● SRPs – ' strange, rare and peculiar' symptoms;
● aetiology;

- mental and intellectual symptoms;
- general symptoms relating to the whole person;
- local symptoms with modalities and/or concomitants.

An essential component in case analysis involves deciding which symptoms are 'useful' in helping the practitioner to choose a remedy to prescribe. Remember that all these techniques are part of the process of pattern recognition. What we are seeking to do here is to see a clear pattern in the patient's story and to match that to a clear pattern in a remedy's story.

As you examine the case history, you should mark the symptoms of quality and then collect them according to the ranking order described above in the context of your understanding of what is happening to the patient (your diagnosis) and what clinical course you expect this illness to take (your prognosis).

The marked useful symptoms may be physically collected on a separate page, in a margin or at the end of the case history. Alternatively, you may 'collect' them simply in your mind. I recommend that it is easier at the outset, and good practice anyway, to collect the symptoms physically rather than purely mentally.

Having collected these symptoms together you may see a clear pattern which makes you think of one or two remedies. This may be on the basis of the 'keynotes' of a remedy being represented in the aetiology or as SRP symptoms. Many people are tempted to prescribe on the basis of one or at most three symptoms which they describe as 'keynotes'. This may be a successful strategy but it is also fraught with danger. Firstly, to what extent are these symptoms keynotes of the remedy? Are they truly characteristic of this remedy? Do they distinguish it from other remedies? Secondly, how important are these symptoms in this particular case? There is a great temptation to see a symptom as 'usable', meaning it makes you think of a remedy, and base your entire prescription on it.

Remember that the closer the match between the patient's symptoms and the features of the remedy, the greater your chances of a good response to the prescription. So, if you do recognize a keynote which brings one particular remedy to mind, you cannot stop there. You have to examine the whole case and examine the picture of the remedy to see how closely they match. This will involve consulting a materia medica. You have to have access to a materia medica if you are going to make intelligent, useful prescriptions.

Often, in acute disease, you will see a striking pattern which you recognize and on the basis of which you will be able to make a good prescription. However, particularly in chronic disease, with its greater complexity, you will not recognize a pattern just by looking at the collected symptoms. This is where the Repertory becomes an essential tool.

What is a 'repertory'?

A repertory is basically a concordance of symptoms. There are several repertories available, but two or three have gained widespread acceptance and are considered as standard. It is impossible for any human to hold in their heads the detailed pictures of over 2000 remedies. These pictures are described, with varying degrees of detail, in the books we call materia medicae. When a patient describes one of their symptoms and you want to know which remedies have that symptom as part of their picture, then the materia medicae are not a great help. Basically, what they lack is a comprehensive index. In essence, the Repertory is a kind of index.

The structure varies between the different repertories, but they all share certain basic features. The chapters of the Repertory each relate to a part of the body or a body system (with some exceptions which will be described below). Each chapter then contains an alphabetically arranged list of symptoms. Each of the symptoms has a list of remedies printed next to it. A symptom with its associated remedies is known as a 'rubric'.

The most widely accepted repertory this century has been *Kent's Repertory*. It has become the standard. However, recent major challenges to this have come from the publications of *Synthesis* and *The Complete Repertory*, both of which have kept the basic structure of Kent. Another modern repertory which has gained a fair degree of support is *Murphy's Repertory*, which has not kept the structure of Kent even to the extent of creating entirely different chapters and presenting the chapters from A to Z rather than in the traditional pattern.

However, despite the publication of these modern works which are fast supplanting Kent, the fact that the two major modern repertories have kept the same structure as Kent makes it worthwhile introducing you to the basics of the layout so that you can begin to find your way around one of these books. The sequence of chapters in this standard format is most easily represented in the form of a table as shown in

Mind	1	Prostate gland	823
Vertigo	213	Urethra	825
Head	225	Urine	837
Eye	359	Male genitalia	849
Vision	399	Female genitalia	879
Ear	415	Larynx/Trachea	927
Hearing	449	Respiration	943
Nose	453	Cough	959
Face	485	Expectoration	991
Mouth	533	Chest	1001
Teeth	569	Back	1065
Throat	587	Extremities	1131
External throat	611	Sleep	1391
Stomach	617	Dreams	1437
Abdomen	683	Chill	1459
Rectum	757	Fever	1477
Stool	789	Perspiration	1491
Bladder	799	Skin	1503
Kidneys	817	Generals	1543

Figure 6.1 The repertory structure developed by Kent and currently used by Schroyens (1993) in *Synthesis*, showing how each chapter relates to a part of the body system.

Figure 6.1. Within a chapter there is an alphabetic sequence of symptoms in headings and subheadings style. There is also a standard sequence of headings and subheadings:

● symptom

● sides

● times

● modalities

● extensions

HOMEOPATHY IN PRIMARY CARE

- localizations
- qualitative description.

This order is adhered to even in the production of subrubrics.

The other main element of the standard formats which applies throughout all the repertories is the use of standard typefaces – normal, italic, bold and capitalized bold (Fig. 6.2). These typefaces correspond to the strength with which the particular remedy has this particular symptom as part of its picture. Traditionally, these typefaces are given a numerical value.

Typeface	Value
normal	1
italic	2
bold	3
CAPITALIZED BOLD	4

Figure 6.2 Typefaces and strengths.

You can see that if you were to go through the whole repertory looking for all the occurrences of a particular remedy and note down the rubrics in which it appeared, you would build a complete picture of that remedy. If you then proceeded to do the same with every remedy you would have reconstructed a materia medica. (I don't recommend it!)

Computer repertories

A number of computerized versions of the repertories are available. These make it much easier to search for a particular symptom or remedy. As well as greatly increasing the speed of repertory analysis (see below), computers make it easy for you to perform multiple and complex analyses to help you look at your case in several different ways (see below).

The uses of the Repertory

A repertory is a tool for working out which remedy the patient needs. This is really both its prime and commonest function. However, it is also a very useful tool for learning about homeopathic remedies.

There are two major challenges for the first-time user of a repertory. In order to find the rubrics which will help you have to know both what words are used and where to find those words. For example, if you wish to look up the symptom 'tearful' or 'crying', you will have to know that, in the Repertory, the rubric is 'weeping'. You also need to know which chapter to consult to find the symptoms related to food likes and dislikes. (In *Synthesis*, this is the 'Generals' chapter.) It is worthwhile browsing through your repertory from time to time just to become familiar with the terminology of the rubrics and their location.

Having found the rubrics which you feel are most representative of your patient's symptoms, the next step is to see whether this process has thrown up the possibility of any remedies which might help this patient. There are various ways to go about this. The simplest is to look in a rubric which you consider to be highly significant in this patient's story. For example, you may be looking at the rubric 'Ailments from anger with indignation'. You can read the remedies listed in this rubric and on the basis of your knowledge of these remedies or by consulting their materia medica descriptions, you may decide that one of them is the appropriate one to prescribe. A step beyond this, is to consider two or three rubrics and see which remedies appear in them, taking particular note of the remedies which appear in all the rubrics you consider. For example, you may look at both the rubrics 'Ailments from anger with indignation' and 'Ailments from anger, suppressed'. Both these methods are often referred to as 'finger repertorizing' (because the practitioner uses a finger to mark the pages where the rubrics appear and then flicks back and forward between them to consider their contents). This is a common method for a practitioner to use during a consultation and may at times provoke the practitioner to ask specific questions to verify or exclude particular remedies which are appearing in the consulted rubrics.

The third method extends this process further and involves noting all the rubrics which are considered relevant and then gathering together the information on the remedies which appear in these rubrics. As we noted earlier, the typeface of the remedy in a rubric is associated with a numerical value. This feature is used in the analysis process. As well as listing all the remedies which appear in the considered rubrics, every time the occurrence of a remedy is noted its numerical value is also noted. This is most easily represented in the form of a grid (Fig. 6.3).

You will see that by listing the remedies as they appear down the first column and marking their numerical value in the column of the rubric, you can then quickly do two things. Firstly, you can see which

HOMEOPATHY IN PRIMARY CARE

Nr	Symptom	Rep	Nr	Symptom	Rep
1					
2					
3					
4					

❶	1 2 3 4 5 6 7 8 S		1 2 3 4 5 6 7 8 S		1 2 3 4 5 6 7 8 S
Acon		Crat-t		Nat-c	
Aesc		Cupr		Nat-m	
Agar				Nat-p	
All-c				Nat-s	
Aloe				Nit-ac	
Alum				Nux-m	
Ambr				Nux-v	
Am-c					
Anac		Dig			
Ant-c		Dros		Olnd	

Figure 6.3 A grid used to analyse the numerical values of remedies.

remedies are appearing in the majority (or even all) of the rubrics considered. Secondly, you can add the ones, twos, threes and fours and produce a total score for each remedy.

It will quickly become obvious to you that this is a slow, laborious process. When done by hand it is also tempting to avoid rubrics which contain a lot of remedies. These inherent drawbacks restrict the usefulness of this method but it is worthwhile analysing a few cases in this way as it gives you a good 'feel' for the process of repertorization.

Using computer repertories

Is there any way to reduce the pain? Yes. The computer-based repertories can analyse your selected rubrics and present you with your table of spread and values in a flash. However, you do trade off one pain for another – in this case the biggest pain is probably financial. All the computer repertories involve buying a computer and a software package costing several hundred pounds. While this does require a significant initial investment they will pay for themselves in the savings of your personal, valuable time very quickly. The computer repertories also make it easier for you to do a variety of examinations of the rubrics. For example, they allow you to weight the symptoms. This is analogous to the underlining we discussed earlier and allows your analysis to take into consideration the relative weightings you have given to the patient's various symptoms. There are many other sophisticated elements in the repertorization process which are possible when using a computer but they are too complex to consider in this text.

Prescribing strategies

There are various ways to consider the case you have taken and each may throw up different potential remedies. Let us look at some of the different ways first and then consider the problem of deciding between them.

Aetiology

If the aetiology is clear and strong it may be possible to find a remedy which is clearly associated with this aetiology, e.g. arnica for ailments from injury which produced significant bruising. Consider the phrase 'never well since. . . .'

Strange, rare or peculiar

Any symptoms of this type which can be translated into rubrics can suggest a small number of remedies.

Keynotes

Three or four keynotes of a remedy in a case will stimulate you to think of that remedy.

Centre of gravity

If the centre of gravity of the case seems to lie clearly in one area, e.g. 'locals' or 'mentals', then the rubrics related to that area may be considered the most appropriate. Remember the hierarchy of the symptoms when assessing the most appropriate centre of gravity.

Family history

This may suggest the presence of a miasm which may lead you to consider remedies consistent with that miasm (see the Appendix for a brief introduction to this subject). Some practitioners use this type of analysis as a working tool. However, I have yet to meet a contemporary leading homeopath who actively uses this approach.

Totality

Using the repertorization processes described above, which remedies best cover the case?

Totality plus sum

Add up the ones, twos, threes and fours in addition to considering the totality.

Potential use of isopathy

Is there a strong allergic basis to this illness? Is it, for example, a simple case of a dog allergy? Is there a clear history of 'never well since' which allows the potential use of a nosode? For example, never well since glandular fever suggests the potential use of glandular fever nosode.

A special kind of isopathy is 'tautopathy'. This refers to the use of a homeopathically prepared remedy made from an allopathic drug, and used to treat a condition which has been caused by that drug. For example, Prednisolone can be used in potentized form to treat ailments from suppression due to Prednisolone. Another use for tautopathy is in the attempt to wean someone off an addiction, e.g. Diazepam.

Some of these strategies require the use of a repertory, some do not. Before taking the next step of choosing between two or more possible strategies I would like to tell you about a couple of other strategies which have emerged in recent years.

One is the consideration of families of remedies. Some remedies have been used extensively and we have an extensive database of knowledge about them. These remedies tend to be well represented in the repertories. Other remedies have been used very infrequently and we have little knowledge of them. Consequently they are poorly represented in the repertories. Considering remedies in 'families' and defining the 'family characteristics' of the remedies is another strategy. For example, maybe many of the features of the remedy Lachesis are represented in the case, but you know from your knowledge and your reading that Lachesis is unlikely to be the correct remedy. Consideration of other snake remedies may lead you to prescribe a lesser known remedy which turns out to be a good remedy for this patient. Dr Massimo Mangialavori of Italy has pioneered this approach and others are working in the same way.

Dr Jan Scholten of The Netherlands has pioneered another strategy drawing upon this original idea of families of remedies and applying it to a study of the elements as represented in the Periodic Table. Jan considers the position of the patient in society and the emotional reaction pattern at the time of becoming ill and develops clear 'themes' of the case from these starting points. These themes can be related to 'periods' or 'stages' (columns) and to 'series' (rows) of the Periodic Table. These ideas are best developed by their original authors.

If there is only one clear prescribing strategy then the relevant remedy will need to be found by using that strategy. However, what happens when there is more than one possible strategy from which to choose? The answer lies partly in clinical experience. The more you practise, the more you will develop an understanding of the relative strengths of the different strategies.

But how do I decide between them? At all times, the best remedy will be the similimum. All the strategies are techniques for suggesting the similimum. Whichever strategy you use, whichever remedy is 'suggested' by your chosen strategy, you must consider whether or not the picture the patient is presenting to you is mirrored in the picture the remedy presents to you. This is the deciding factor.

If you are still stuck, then use the rules of symptom analysis, including the hierarchy of symptoms described above, to choose a strategy for your first prescription.

Key points

- Your first goal is to understand the patient.
- Your second goal is to decide whether or not you consider it appropriate to prescribe a homeopathic remedy.
- Your third goal is to work out which remedy you wish to prescribe.
- The symptoms which have the greatest importance are the 'strange, rare, peculiar' symptoms.

CHOOSING A DOSAGE REGIME

7

The dosage regime consists of two elements – the potency and the frequency of dosing.

By this stage you will have decided which particular remedy or remedies you are going to prescribe. The choice of potency should be guided by the rules described in Chapter 4. Do not get hung up on this point. The selection of the remedy is far more important than the choice of the potency.

Frequency of dosing can best be summarized as follows – repeat the remedy once its effect has worn off. In acute disease this may result in very frequent dosing, e.g. every 15 minutes or so initially. In chronic disease it may result in very infrequent dosing, e.g. once every few months. Many practitioners give a single dose, then wait until follow-up. Others give a 'split single dose' of three doses spread over 24 hours or over 3 days. The thinking behind this regime is to reduce the incidence of aggravations and to increase the chances of a successful 'hit' from the remedy.

Non-classical prescribers may give a dose of the remedy twice a day on a continuing basis until symptoms disappear. Others use sac lac as a placebo drug on an ongoing basis. For example, they may give 30 doses to be taken one dose a day for 30 days. Only the first 1–3 doses contain the active remedy; the rest are simply sac lac (sac lac is the transport medium on which the remedies are carried).

The arguments in favour of this approach are that patients want to take something every day and cannot understand the concept of only taking a single dose. My own experience is directly counter to this. I have found that taking the time to explain why I am only giving one dose of a remedy is always worthwhile. I think it also empowers the patient and helps them to understand that the healing which they are undergoing is essentially the healing of their own systems, not an artificial healing dependent on the effect of a drug. I have never prescribed sac lac.

Key point

● Only repeat the remedy once its effect has worn off.

FOLLOW-UP: WHAT HAS HAPPENED? 8

The follow-up consultation presents a new set of challenges to the practitioner. Has the remedy worked? What am I going to do now? These are the dominant questions in the practitioner's mind.

I have seen numerous complex and complicated attempts to guide students through this difficult task. Let us keep the approach simple and direct.

Your first question to yourself should be: change or no change? Simply, has any change occurred since the last visit?

If there is really no change then what can this mean? The possibilities are as follows.

Wrong remedy

The prescribed remedy did nothing because it was not the appropriate remedy. This is usually our first thought, largely because of our lack of confidence in our abilities to choose the right remedies first time.

However, it is not necessarily the correct conclusion. Re-take the case. Is there other significant information which you missed last time? How confident are you that the remedy prescribed was the right remedy? Consider the other possible explanations for there being no change.

Obstacle to cure

The concept of obstacles to cure is an interesting one and is, I think, unique to the practice of homeopathy. The idea is that the remedy given is well chosen and the practitioner is reasonably expecting to see a change, but a change has failed to occur, so maybe something in the patient's life has 'blocked' the expected effect of the remedy.

What kinds of things can block the effect of a remedy? Hahnemann described a large number of possibilities in his Organon. In effect, they all belong to one of three categories.

Medicines

Any medicines can potentially adversely affect the action of a remedy. The most notorious classes of drug are the immunosuppressants and antiinflammatories, particularly steroids. It is interesting that this class has been most frequently implicated, as the immune system and the inflammatory system can be thought of as essential parts of the body's healing mechanism – the very healing capacity which remedies hope to stimulate. However, there are sporadic reports of many classes of medicine having such adverse effects. In perspective, it should be said that patients who require these drugs can still respond favourably to a homeopathic remedy. The homeopathic hospitals, for example, routinely treat people with serious, disabling conditions without requiring them to stop their life-saving drugs.

Medicinal substances in diet or atmosphere

This includes any chemical or biochemical substance in the environment which can exert a biological effect on humans. Tobacco smoke, alcohol, caffeine, fumes, etc. are examples.

Excesses

Hahnemann's third category is excesses of living. Much of this looks moralistic, but mostly it is just common sense, in relation to excesses of sexual behaviour, diet, stress and domestic hygiene.

A special category, related to obstacle to cure, is the 'exciting cause'. By this we mean that if some external provoking 'cause' for the patient's illness can be identified, then this cause should be removed. For example, if the patient has a gluten enteropathy, then gluten must be excluded from the diet.

HOMEOPATHY IN PRIMARY CARE

Wrong potency

The remedy seems to be chosen well and still looks like the one best indicated. There are no obvious obstacles to cure, yet the remedy has failed to act. It could be the potency choice is to blame. The remedy should be repeated but in a different potency or even in a range of potencies (some prescribers would give the remedy in three doses with ascending potency, e.g. 30c followed by a dose of 200c, followed by a dose of 1M).

This is probably much less likely than a 'wrong remedy' or 'obstacle to cure' reason.

Inactive remedy

The remedy prescribed was 'dud'. This explanation is usually favoured by a more experienced prescriber who is convinced of his or her own homeopathic skill, feels the remedy prescribed was well indicated and given in an appropriate potency and there are no significant obstacles to cure. Therefore, in the face of no response, the most likely explanation was that the particular batch prescribed was inactive. Thoughts of a bad workman blaming his tools are bound to arise, but this may, indeed, be the correct explanation. Simple repetition of the prescription, dispensed from a different batch, is the only possible action in this case.

So, what if there has been change since the last visit? This scenario is a bit more complicated than the 'no change' one. However, let us examine the possibilities.

I think there are only three possible changes.

1. better
2. worse
3. mixed.

In all cases of change it is important to first check and see exactly what changes there have been. It is important, therefore, to consult your records of the patient's previous visits. The opening remarks of a patient in follow-up are often fairly unhelpful, e.g. 'Fine' or 'No better' or 'Worse'. You should methodically check to see which symptoms are better or worse, what has happened to the patient's well-being, energy levels and emotional state.

If there is amelioration of all the main symptoms, improvement in mood, energy and well-being, then all is progressing well. In this situation you should leave well alone. There is no indication to repeat a remedy if the patient is improving at a satisfactory speed.

Has the patient developed any new symptoms since the last visit? If they have, then what is the significance of these new symptoms? Do they represent a progression of the pathology? In other words, are they symptoms you would expect with this diagnosis if the illness were to progress?

Are the symptoms an 'aggravation'? The phenomenon of the aggravation causes much debate in homeopathic circles. Some practitioners claim to see it rarely, others claim to see it every time they prescribe. Everyone agrees that patients who experience an aggravation are most likely to experience a deep and lasting amelioration of their condition. Many practitioners, indeed, feel much more comfortable with their choice of remedy if the patient has experienced an aggravation.

So what is an aggravation? It is a temporary exacerbation of the existing symptoms. It is thought to be the primary action of the remedy – the first response of the healing process. It should occur very soon after the remedy is taken and a so-called aggravation appearing several days or weeks after the remedy is taken is probably not an aggravation at all. Typically aggravations are not severe or long-lasting. Their appearance is a good sign, the patient should be reassured and no treatment should be given. However, if the aggravation is causing distressing symptoms then it may need to be treated. It is commonly held that in this circumstance it is best to use an allopathic treatment rather than a homeopathic one. Treatment of an aggravation carries with it the risk of suppression and, thereby, reversal of the healing which is underway. Do your best to leave well alone.

Aggravations should only involve symptoms which are not new to the patient. They may be existing symptoms or symptoms consistent with the direction of cure.

If there are new symptoms which are not consistent with the pathology of the disease, not consistent with direction of cure and are part of the remedy picture, then they are probably a proving. The case should be reassessed and a different remedy will probably be indicated.

HOMEOPATHY IN PRIMARY CARE

Key points

- Obstacles to cure – medicines, medicinal substances in the diet and excesses.
- An aggravation is a temporary exacerbation of the existing symptoms.

ASSESSING OUTCOME

9

It is very useful to assess the outcome of your homeopathic treatment. Firstly, it enables you to make sensible decisions about further management. Secondly, it helps you to learn lessons about your own work – where your strengths and weaknesses lie. Thirdly, it helps you learn about remedies (by studying the cases of 'cured' patients). Fourthly, it helps you and others to make convincing arguments for increasing the availability of homeopathy as a therapeutic modality.

Ways of assessing outcome

You can assess use of other health care interventions by recording allopathic drug usage before and after treatment, by assessing hospital outpatient and inpatient attendances, investigations and procedures carried out before and after treatment and by assessing use of primary care services before and after treatment. You can also use one of the clinical outcome scores in use.

I would like to bring to your attention an outcome score developed and used in Scotland currently and to show you how you could use this method in your own practice without having to reinvent the wheel.

The Glasgow Homoeopathic Hospital has developed a standard audit score based on a 0–4 (plus or minus) scale related to changes in the patient's life, using words with which the patient can identify.

The score is as follows:

 0 No change
+1 Slight improvement, not sufficient to affect daily living
+2 Moderate improvement, sufficient to affect daily living
+3 Major improvement
+4 Complete resolution, cure.

In terms of deterioration the scale mirrors the positives of the improvement, thus

 0 No change
−1 Slight deterioration, not sufficient to affect daily living
−2 Moderate deterioration, sufficient to affect daily living
−3 Major deterioration
−4 Disastrous deterioration.

The scale can be applied to one or more specific symptoms of the patient and/or to well-being.

The International Data Collection Unit at the Glasgow Homoeopathic Hospital will provide further information about this scale and the current international projects being carried out using it. If you wish to be involved in this work then write to: The Data Collection Unit, Glasgow Homoeopathic Hospital, 1000 Great Western Road, Glasgow G12 0NR, Scotland, UK.

THE COMMON QUESTIONS

Introduction

There are several questions which arise with great frequency when health care professionals begin to practise homeopathy in the primary care setting. Many of these issues are common to all workers in this field and these are addressed below. There are also some specific issues of relevance to particular primary care professionals and these will be addressed after this section.

How can homeopathy be integrated into the primary care team?

The first question to be answered is 'Who is a member of the primary care team?' The answer is different in different countries.

Let us define primary care as 'first contact care'. The members of the team are, therefore, those health care workers who are the first contact for individuals who seek health care. This still brings different answers in different countries and in all countries the primary care team itself is under constant review and change. In all countries, the family doctor or general practitioner tends to be regarded as the key player in the primary care team. In the UK, the average team would also have community nurses and practice nurses, midwives and health visitors as members. Beyond this, teams may include members of other professions allied to medicine (as defined in UK law), plus secretarial and administrative support.

In the US primary care teams are unlikely to include midwives or health visitors and may typically have nurse practitioners and/or physician's assistants as members. There are also a greater number of doctors considered as primary care doctors in the US – particularly paediatricians, obstetrician/gynaecologists and internists.

Primary care workers, particularly family doctors, tend to have continuity of care of their patients through various stages of their lives and are therefore ideally placed to consider their patients from a holistic perspective. However, sheer pressure of work combined with lack of available time produces real and stressful constraints on practitioner and patient alike. Learning about homeopathy can widen the range of therapeutic possibilities open to the primary care professional but it can also bring some additional stresses. The purpose of this section of the book is to look at some of the practicalities of homeopathic practice within a primary care setting.

How long does a homeopathic consultation take?

How long is a piece of string? There is, of course, no simple answer to this question as there are many factors to take into consideration. Acute disease can be dealt with more quickly than chronic disease. How much information does the practitioner have before the consultation begins? How much experience does the practitioner have?

However, a basic rule of thumb is that an acute homeopathic consultation should not take significantly more time than a non-homeopathic one. The use of homeopathy in the acute primary care setting has no significant impact on consultation times and can therefore be introduced without major changes in the appointment system. (I am assuming the standard 10-minute appointment. If your appointment slots are less than 10 minutes apart, you are probably going to find it difficult to deal with acute problems effectively, whether or not you are using homeopathy.)

To take a full homeopathic history, which will be necessary if you wish to deal with chronic problems, will take about 1 hour. It is very difficult to have a good, full, homeopathic consultation in less than 1 hour and many practitioners allow $1\frac{1}{2}$ hours. However, note that this is the time required to conduct the consultation and you may need to do the case analysis, repertorization and prescribing outwith this time in most cases. Cutting corners on this will produce poorer results and decrease both patient and professional satisfaction. If you cannot find this time in your working week, then it is probably best to refer all patients requiring this amount of involvement to a homeopathic specialist.

How often does a patient have to attend?

Again, there are lots of 'depends' in this answer. In the treatment of acute problems, the patient does not have to attend any more frequently than you would otherwise plan. In fact, if they are being treated more effectively, then they may attend even less frequently than expected. However, in the early stages of your homeopathic practice, you will be keen to see what results you achieve. (I hope you will retain this desire well beyond the initial weeks and months. Audit can become seamless and routine if it is conducted in a manner which is not time-consuming.) You may initially, therefore, find yourself asking more patients with acute, self-limiting complaints back for review than you would do otherwise. There are, however, no specific homeopathic reasons to increase your 'return rate'.

In the management of chronic diseases an average number of visits is eight per year. Beyond that, the practitioner should be carefully reviewing the course of the case to judge whether or not progress is being made with this approach. He or she may decide at this point that a different therapeutic avenue be pursued.

What is the likely impact on appointment availability of introducing homeopathy?

From the consideration of the average consultation time and the frequency of review, it should be possible to make some estimate of the overall effects on appointment availability. The enticing ideal, of course, is that the homeopathic interventions are more effective than the current treatment approaches so more patients get better more quickly. This ideal would increase appointment availability. Other factors which may actually increase appointment availability are the practice of homeopathy by a wider range of members of the primary care team than just the doctors and patient education in homeopathic self-care.

If your use of homeopathy is restricted to management of acute disease with referral of any more complex or chronic problems to a homeopathic specialist, then there will be little adverse impact on appointment availability. The more you begin to take full homeopathic histories and manage a greater number of chronic and complex problems yourself, the more you will find an adverse effect on appointment availability. A full homeopathic history in a patient with a complex and/or chronic problem takes at least an hour. Follow-up appointments will take at least 20 minutes. If an average number of return visits over the course of a year is seven, then you are working with a new:return visit ratio of 1:7. A full homeopathic session with one new and seven return patients would take 200 minutes. If your normal booking interval is 10 minutes, this means you could have seen 20 patients in the time taken to do the homeopathic session where you saw eight patients. Clearly, this has a big impact on appointment availability. An understanding of this can be useful in determining how much you are willing to take on at this level. One new patient a week? One new patient a month?

How can I find time for longer consultations?

As already stated, homeopathic management of all but the acute diseases requires fuller case taking and case analysis. This requires longer consultations. There are basically three approaches to finding the time for these longer consultations.

1. Setting aside 'special' time in the form of an evening consultation or a half-day when you would otherwise not be working.

2. Setting aside 'special' time at the end or the beginning of routine appointment sessions.

3. Integrated into the routine appointment sessions. If a normal appointment is 10 minutes, then a double appointment is sufficient time for a homeopathic follow-up and three double appointments spread over a few days or weeks is sufficient time for a full homeopathic history. One way of following this approach is to spend the first appointment taking only the presenting history, the second appointment concentrating on the homeopathic 'generals' area (and filling in any background which you do not already have – past medical history, family history, etc.) and the third appointment concentrating on the 'mentals'.

Which of these three approaches works for you will depend on your current routine and the overall work of your full primary care team.

Where should I record the history?

The question is whether to integrate the homeopathic information with the patient medical record or maintain a separate record for homeopathic interventions. It would seem better practice to integrate. We do not have a tradition of using separate record sheets for separate treatment modalities. However, if you are working as a member of a team, this case has to be fully accepted by all team members. Other team members will then be aware that some of your entries are much longer than the 'regular' ones, but prior explanation should prevent this from being a problem.

In terms of integration, two different approaches have emerged. One is full integration, with the homeopathic history being entered in the standard record in the routine manner. The second is writing the homeopathic information on separate sheets which are filed in their own section within the standard record. This latter approach has a number of advantages. The whole homeopathic history, if built up gradually over time, can still be read as a unitary whole and 'homeopathic observations' can be added at any time. For example, during a visit to the patient's house you may notice that they are extremely neat and tidy. You might note in the relevant homeopathic section 'fastidious'. Other observations gleaned can be recorded in this manner, building up a picture of the patient over time. This information may then be useful to you if you ever set out to deal with a complex or chronic problem homeopathically.

There are also certain techniques of recording the history which may be enhanced by a slightly different page layout from the routine one. The use of a fairly wide margin is one example. This allows note to be made of possible remedies as the history is given. For example, if the patient mentions that all their pains have a burning quality and they ease them by applying hot wraps, then the practitioner might record Arsenicum Album in the margin at this point.

Other recording techniques within the case history include starring important symptoms with an asterisk, and underlining according to the principles of intensity, spontaneity and clarity. There are other recording techniques which aid case analysis and for which space has to be made available. These include listing the rubrics chosen, perhaps including a computer-generated repertorization, listing the reasons for the choice of the remedy given and using some standard audit sheet to facilitate assessment of outcome.

Are there any shortcuts to history taking?

The one big potential advantage to having more than one primary care team member trained in the homeopathic approach is that the homeopathic history taking can be shared. This may happen in both formal and informal ways. It may be a deliberate policy to have part of the history taken by one primary care team member before the full analysis is performed and a prescription issued. This is very similar to the model of antenatal clinics in the UK, where a midwife takes the woman's history and performs the initial examination and then an obstetrician reviews the information, focuses on certain areas with the patient and draws up a management plan with the midwife. Having a clearly separate homeopathic history recording sheet is an aid to this process and such a sheet may have a structure which aids history taking.

Others use questionnaires in this process as a shortcut. Different ways of using such an aid have been tried, including having the patient fill in the details unaided at home before attending the practitioner or, alternatively, having someone with homeopathic training guide them through the process. Only a minority of practitioners remain enthusiastic about questionnaires after using them for a while. They tend to be restrictive and mechanical, reducing the history taking to a data collection task. This is only likely, however, if the questionnaire is used as a substitute for a consultation.

Should I repertorize during a consultation?

Our training places heavy emphasis on memory. To consult textbooks during a consultation, in front of a patient, is thought to damage the patient's confidence in the practitioner and to suggest a disturbing lack of knowledge. However, as there are over 2000 possible remedies and the patient requires a remedy individually chosen for them, the chances of the practitioner being able to pick the right remedy without consulting a book are slim. It is the mark of a good practitioner to consult a repertory during the consultation. If this causes you some difficulty initially, explicit explanations to your patients may make you more comfortable. Usually patients are quite fascinated by the Repertory and giving them some insight into the homeopathic process enhances the relationship with them. The greatest value from using the Repertory during the consultation is that as rubrics cast up possible remedies, relevant questions can be asked to confirm or exclude the possibilities.

HOMEOPATHY IN PRIMARY CARE

What about other homeopathic books, such as clinical compendia and materia medicae?

Clinical compendia look as if they would be useful books to consult during a consultation, but practitioners rarely seem to find them so. However, in the early stages of your practice they may prove useful. Materia medicae are basic reference texts and you will want to consult them regularly. They do not, however, offer ideas for possible remedies. Consequently, their greatest value is usually at the stage of case analysis which may be done following the consultation.

Will I be tempted to prescribe remedies for self-limiting diseases?

Yes you probably will, particularly when presented with a 'strange, rare or peculiar' symptom or a clear, well-established indication. Whether or not you do prescribe even when you can think of a remedy depends on your attitude to patient empowerment and work demand. You are unlikely to want to become known as the person with the remedies for minor colds, sore throats, etc. Such a reputation risks your being inundated! It is also widely regarded as good practice not to encourage a mentality of 'a pill for every ill'. The body has remarkable healing powers. You must ask yourself both 'What is the value of my prescription?' and 'What will be the consequences for this patient of my intervention?'. Such consultations may, however, usefully provide opportunities for patient education and thereby patient empowerment.

How do I address patients' issues?

Certain questions arise frequently when a patient attends for his or her first homeopathic consultation. Here are a few of them, with suggested answers.

Why are you asking me these strange questions?

I need to understand you and how this illness affects your life. Everyone who has the same diagnosis as you is a unique person and though they have the same diagnosis, the actual symptoms which they experience may be markedly different from yours. These differences are important to help me establish the unique nature of your experience. (The patient is most likely to find the questions relating to the 'generals' odd. This may be tackled as follows.)

I am now going to ask you some questions about yourself. These questions help me to find out how you are affected by various environmental influences. They help me to understand your 'physiology'.

Why do I not have to take a tablet every day or even several times a day? How can so few doses have any effect?

Medicines like painkillers suppress the body's symptoms. Homeopathic remedies work by stimulating your own self-healing and self-repairing systems. They are not suppressing anything so don't have to be taken frequently. Remember when you were immunized against polio? You received a few drops of the polio vaccine on your tongue. The doctor did not give you a huge bottle of polio vaccine and tell you to take three spoonsful a day for the rest of your life. That was because the polio vaccine worked by stimulating your body's own defence mechanisms – the immune system. The remedies are also stimulating, not suppressive.

Another analogy is the one of the grandfather clock with a pendulum. To get it going again you do not have to push the pendulum every second but, instead, you push the pendulum once and then wait till it stops again before giving it another push.

Are you giving me tablets which have nothing in them?

Whilst it is true that many of the substances we use as homeopathic remedies are very poisonous in their raw form, they have been subjected to a process which removes the poisonous molecules but actually enhances the healing potential of the original substances. So, as the remedies do have healing potential and we repeatedly see that only the right remedy for you will have the hoped – for healing effect, it is not true to say they have 'nothing' in them.

HOMEOPATHY IN PRIMARY CARE

How should I store the remedies?

Most medicines are fairly delicate and need to be treated quite carefully. Homeopathic remedies should be stored away from strong light, strong temperature variations and strong smells. All three can inactivate them.

Does that mean I cannot use homeopathy and aromatherapy at the same time?

You should not store your homeopathic remedies in the same place as your aromatherapy oils and you should not take a homeopathic remedy at exactly the same time as you apply an aromatherapy oil, but you can undergo both treatments for your illness.

How should I handle the remedies?

As little as possible. Try to touch them with your fingers only if you really have to and as little as you can. Handling the remedies too much can inactivate them.

Should I stop my other medication?

No. Homeopathic remedies can be safely taken along with other medicines. It can be very dangerous to suddenly stop a medicine which you have been using for some time. The remedies will not interfere with your other drugs. You will be able to reduce your other drugs if you begin to improve under the influence of the homeopathic ones.

So why have I heard that some homeopaths tell their patients to stop their other drugs?

It is very unusual for a qualified health care professional to give such an instruction. Some non-medically qualified homeopaths have been known to give such advice and it stems from their distrust of mainstream medicine. The reason they will give is that some drugs can inhibit the effects of the homeopathic remedies. It is true that some drugs can produce such an inhibitory effect, particularly steroids and other drugs which suppress the immune system. However, experienced homeopathic practitioners will tell you that it is still possible for the remedies to produce good effects in the face of these drugs. Drugs should only be stopped when it is deemed they are no longer clinically necessary.

What other things can prevent a remedy from acting?

Several external influences may inhibit the action of a remedy. The ingestion of strong stimulants such as coffee, alcohol, nicotine and recreational drugs. A bad dose of an infectious disease like influenza or food poisoning. A shock or emotional trauma. The continued influence of the primary aetiological factor. Other drugs or treatments.

However, we must not forget that everyone is an individual and if the response to the remedy is not as good as hoped, then we should see whether or not anything in the environment may be having an adverse effect.

Patient information leaflets

Many practitioners find it helpful to have an information leaflet covering some of the above points available for their patients to take away and read.

What are the cost implications of the service?

Savings

Potential savings are possible in both the drug bill and the purchase of other medical and surgical interventions. There is also a potential saving in the purchase of investigations as the homeopathic method enhances clinical skills of history taking and observation.

Income

Homeopathy is becoming increasingly popular and the increased demand brings financial rewards to those who can respond to that demand.

Expenditure

The biggest expenditure is on training the practitioner, a process which should continue throughout his or her working life. This mainly consists of attending educational courses and purchasing textbooks. The remedies themselves are extremely inexpensive. There are no investigations to purchase. The other potential expenditure is on a computer-based repertory and this is optional.

Obtaining remedies for patients

Most homeopathic practitioners personally dispense remedies to patients, either directly from stock or indirectly, after obtaining the remedy on the patient's behalf from a homeopathic pharmaceutical manufacturer.

Most homeopathic remedies can be purchased directly and homeopathic pharmaceutical manufacturers are usually happy to supply the relevant remedy directly to the patient if the patient sends the prescription to the company. In the UK, homeopathy is and has always been an integral part of the NHS. Homeopathic prescriptions can therefore be written on standard NHS prescription forms and dispensed by the local pharmacy.

Many local pharmacies are more than happy to stock homeopathic remedies as it increases the number of customers coming to their shop. Some pharmacies become particularly interested, send their pharmacists on training courses and build up large stocks of remedies.

Dealing with colleagues

Other members of the primary care team

The reactions of your colleagues to your new homeopathic skills will range from fascination through indifference to downright hostility. All three reactions can be troublesome, but especially the two extremes. Your colleagues may start to refer to you all their own 'heartsink' patients and all the most difficult clinical problems which they have been unable to resolve. Remember this is a new skill for you. It is not fair to either you or your patients for you to attempt to succeed where everyone else has failed. Just say 'no' to strangers. Don't accept your colleagues' greatest challenges. Explain that you are just starting out and that you don't feel you have the necessary skill or experience in the subject to deal with the most difficult cases. However, your colleagues may wish to refer some of these patients to a qualified, experienced homeopathic specialist.

Indifference can be very demoralizing. Primary care medicine can be a very lonely, isolated pursuit. If your colleagues are indifferent you will benefit from the support of other like-minded individuals in your area. Maybe your national homeopathic organization can put you in touch with such colleagues.

In fact, when your colleagues are downright hostile you also need a lot of support. Careful audit of your work, openness and recognition of your own limitations can go a long way to reducing hostility. Make sure you can, at least, get their agreement to value your clinical freedom as much as their own and to act professionally by not voicing their hostility to patients. If you cannot secure this, then you are probably in serious difficulties anyway, irrespective of whether or not you practise homeopathy. Tell your colleagues about your 'successes', share your clinical audit with them. Study the impact of your use of homeopathy on other aspects of the workload and the profits of the business.

What about other specialists?

Consultant colleagues who know nothing about homeopathy will also demonstrate the full range of reactions to the subject. Should you mention the homeopathic treatment when referring a patient to a consultant colleague? It is probably useful to do so, although not in any great detail. It may stimulate some interest and it may generate comment, either directly or via the patient, which will make it clear which specialists are sympathetic and which are not. This may guide your future referral decisions.

Remember that if you are the family physician, you retain overall responsibility for the patient's welfare. The specialist sees the patient on your behalf. If he or she is rude or dismissive, you can refer to someone else in future.

What about homeopathically trained colleagues?

If you refer to a homeopathic specialist it is particularly helpful to present the salient features of the history, the remedies prescribed and the reactions to them. You should also make clear the extent to which you wish to be involved in ongoing homeopathic care of the patient. It may be that the specialist can share the care with you.

All the advice given in this chapter is of relevance to all health care professionals who wish to practise homeopathy. However, there are some other issues to consider if you are not a doctor.

Practising within the limits of your professional discipline

You should always practise homeopathy within the limits of your own discipline. If you are a chiropodist you will not be expected to use your homeopathic skill to treat gynaecological problems, for example. Homeopathy can add value to your work whatever your professional discipline within the primary care team. Ethically and professionally, you will be judged by your peers and your clinical actions should always aim at the highest standards of your discipline.

Practising with the support of your seniors

It is vital for your own professional safety that you practise your homeopathic skills openly with the support of your seniors to whom you are responsible. The ideal position is to be working with a doctor who at least supports the practice of homeopathy and at best actually practises it personally. You can evolve a good, mutually supportive relationship if there is more than one member of the primary care team involved in homeopathy (ideally, with one of them being a doctor).

Supervision

Homeopathy is not a skill you'll acquire in a weekend or two. It is a lifelong study which grows from dedicated practice. It is essential to get some kind of clinical supervision. Hopefully, your training organization can give you this. However, if they cannot, you should try to become involved with a local group of practitioners or even make a personal arrangement for a homeopathic specialist to provide you with some clinical supervision.

Your knowledge and understanding of homeopathy will grow over the years. It will grow most readily if done in association with like-minded colleagues. This is one of the benefits of two or more members of the same primary care team learning and practising homeopathy.

COMMON CLINICAL INDICATIONS FOR HOMEOPATHY IN PRIMARY HEALTH CARE

Introduction

This section has information about useful remedies for a wide range of commonly encountered clinical conditions. There are four main subsections:

1. No effective allopathic treatment
2. Unsafe situation for allopathic treatment
3. Unacceptable side-effect profile
4. Reduction of allopathic treatment.

As you broaden and deepen your homeopathic skills, you will feel confident to prescribe in more situations.

The first subsection, 'No effective allopathic treatment', covers many of the easiest areas for prescribing homeopathy. Conversely, the fourth subsection, 'Reduction of allopathic treatment', covers some of the most difficult areas.

This textbook is an introductory one. Therefore, for each of the clinical conditions, only between one and three remedies will be described. The description of the remedies follows the format of the Materia Medica information given in Section 4.

In this text, the description of the remedies is of 'Level 1' (a striking characteristic or well-established indication of the remedy), 'Level 2' (the remedy keynotes, including major modalities) and, where appropriate, 'Level 3' (condensed Materia Medica) information relevant to the clinical condition under discussion. The descriptions are deliberately brief and the number of remedies given for each condition is small.

In all cases, the pattern of symptoms shown by this individual patient has to be closely matched by the remedy prescribed. This section is not intended to encourage you to prescribe 'pathologically'. There is no single 'remedy for xxxx' and at all times, homeopathy works best when the treatment is individualized. However, we all need to begin somewhere. Being overwhelmed with too much information about too many remedies is a common cause of practitioners giving up in the early days of their practice.

The remedies described in the following pages are not necessarily the 'best' remedies in these clinical conditions. Indeed, there is a dearth of research to show which remedies are more frequently successful in particular conditions. Instead, the remedies have clear prescribing features which are seen commonly in these clinical conditions.

If your patient with, for example, an anal fissure is complaining of symptoms very similar to the characteristics of one of the described remedies, then prescribe that remedy. If, however, your patient's symptoms do not seem to match the descriptions of any of the remedies presented here, then he or she probably requires a different remedy. In this latter situation, you can either simply do what you would normally do for any patient with this condition and rule out homeopathy as a treatment option in this case or set aside more time with the patient to take a fuller history and try to work out the remedy for yourself. Alternatively, you may choose to refer this patient to a homeopathic specialist.

If the remedy you choose does not help the patient, do not despair as the success of prescribing on the basis of a small number of key-notes is limited. You may have to set aside more time to understand your patient's illness more fully and gain a fuller picture before you can 'discover' the remedy your patient needs or you may decide it is best to enlist the help of a homeopathic specialist at this point.

Note: The conventional symbols of < and >, representing 'worse with' and 'better with' respectively, will be used throughout this section.

NO EFFECTIVE ALLOPATHIC TREATMENT

Allergies

Isopathy

Any allergen can be potentized and used to desensitize a patient. Amongst the more commonly used substances are house dust mite and mixed grass pollens. The decision about which allergen to use can be based on either the history alone or on a combination of the history and the results of allergy tests, such as skin tests or RAST tests.

Different practitioners have used different treatment regimes to treat allergies in this way. The most common regime is to give three doses of a 30c or 200c potency over 1–3 days. This regime is then repeated at monthly intervals until the desensitization has been achieved.

The commonest alternative to this is to treat the patient with a 30c of the remedy twice daily during the time of exposure to the allergen, e.g. through the pollen season in the case of hay fever.

Urtica Urens

Urticarial skin eruptions < bathing; warmth; violent exercise.

Allium Cepa

Perennial rhinitis. Hay fever. Excoriating nasal discharge with bland lachrymation.

Allergies

Isopathy
Urtica Urens
Allium Cepa

> **Case history**
> 12-year-old boy with 'a cold all the time'. Gives a story of runny nose and sneezing every day. Worse at the start of the day. No seasonal variation. Mum also notes he sneezes uncontrollably if he helps her change bedclothes. Skin test confirms allergy to house dust mite.
> *Treatment*:   house dust mite 200c, one dose three times in 24 hours.

Anal Fissure

Nitricum Acidum

Pains sticking like splinters < touch. Anxiety about health.

Silica

Chronic fissure, slow to heal, < cold.

Graphites

Smarting, itching around anus. Cutting pain during defaecation followed by constriction and aching for several hours.

Case history

40-year-old man with sharp sticking pain in the anus. Worse on defaecation and worse when touched. Very sensitive individual who eats the fat which others leave at dinner. Attends the doctor frequently with worries about his health. Examination confirms anal fissure.

Treatment: Nitricum Acidum 200c, one dose three times in 24 hours.

Anger

Nux Vomica

Anger and impatience in hard-working, hard-living individuals who are fastidious and crave stimulants.

Staphysagria

Ailments from suppressed anger with indignation. 'Sweet' individuals who feel they have been unfairly treated and suppress their anger.

Hepar Sulphuris Calcareum

Violent rage leading to violent deeds. Hurried, oversensitive individuals who tend to contradict others.

Case history

35-year-old business executive. Smoker. Hardworking. Very particular and tidy. Extremely irritable, with slamming of doors and banging down the telephone at work.

Treatment: Nux Vomica 200c, one dose, three times over 24 hours.

Chickenpox

Herpes Zoster
Nosode
Rhus
Toxicodendron
Mezereum

Chickenpox

Herpes Zoster Nosode

Can be used as a single dose at the onset of the chickenpox. Also useful where recovery is slow or the patient has never been well since the chickenpox.

Rhus Toxicodendron

Urticaria, vesicles. Least cold air makes skin painful. Restless. > movement, < cold, damp.

Mezereum

Eruptions ulcerate and form thick scabs under which purulent matter exudes. Painful eruptions, sensitive to cold.

Case history

4-year-old girl with chickenpox of 6 days onset. The eruptions are thickly scabbed and painful to touch. Some have become infected and are oozing pus. The eruptions are particularly sensitive to cold air.

Treatment: Mezereum 30c three times daily until healing is under way.

Chilblains

Agaricus Muscarius

Very sensitive to cold. Stitching, splinter-like pains.

Petroleum

When skin is broken, e.g. cracks on fingertips, especially in winter months.

Zincum Metallicum

< rubbing and touch. Restless, fidgety feet.

Colic

Colocynthis

Severe sudden cramping pain > firm pressure.

Magnesia Phosphorica

Cramping abdominal pain making patient bend double, > hot applications.

Stannum Metallicum

Pains which come and go gradually, > rapid motion.

Case history

3-month-old child in good health but every evening she becomes very distressed with screaming and pulling up her legs. Seems to settle a bit if carried with tummy lying on Mum's supporting hand.

Treatment: Colocynthis 30c granules every 15 minutes during colic until it settles.

Fears and phobias

Fears and
phobias

Argentum
Nitricum

Gelsemium

Phosphoricum
Acidum

Argentum Nitricum

Anticipation anxiety with diarrhoea and flatulence.

Gelsemium

Stage fright. Anticipatory anxiety. Paralysis of mind, voice or body.

Phosphoricum Acidum

Many fears – fears something will happen, imaginary things, insanity, dark, thunderstorms.

Case history

70-year-old woman. Housebound because every time she tries to go out to the shops she gets diarrhoea and desperately has to run to the toilet. Lots of gurgling noise in tummy. Feels very anxious and panicky. Craves sweet things.

Treatment: Argentum Nitricum 10M, one as required for the anxiety and diarrhoea.

Gall bladder colic

Berberis Vulgaris

Biliary and renal calculi. Pains rapidly changing character and locality.
Pains radiating out from one point.

Calcarea Carbonica

Overweight, cold, flatulent and sweaty. < cold, pressure of clothes,
milk.

Chelidonium Majus

Jaundice. Icterus. Biliary disorders. Liver pains radiating backward.

Glandular fever

Glandular Fever Nosode

Of use after confirmation of diagnosis. Single dose given during the illness may reduce both the duration and severity of the illness. Similarly, a single dose is indicated in those who have 'never been well since' glandular fever illness.

Belladonna

In the acute stage of the disease when the fever is still present. Indicated when onset is sudden.

Calcarea Phosphorica

Glandular swellings. Coldness or soreness in spots. Craves ham, bacon or smoked meat.

Case history

18-year-old female student who has never been well since contracting glandular fever, confirmed with blood tests 8 months ago. Symptoms vague and non-specific. Weariness, poor concentration interfering with studies.

Treatment: Glandular fever nosode 200c, one dose three times over 24 hours.

Grief

Ignatia

Silent grief. Sighing.

Natrum Muriaticum

Weeps alone. Consolation aggravates. Ailments from grief.

Causticum

Ailments from long-lasting grief. Intensely sympathetic individuals who weep at least trifle.

Case history

65-year-old woman. Sad and withdrawn since death of husband a year ago. Recurrent headaches since his death. Cannot bear direct sunlight without a hat. Does not like fuss and hates it when people show her sympathy. Does not cry easily, but cries alone at home.

Treatment: Natrum Muriaticum 10M, one dose.

HOMEOPATHY IN PRIMARY CARE

Impotence

Lycopodium

Lack of confidence. Apprehension. Desire to be in control.

Conium

Stopping and starting of urinary flow.

Phosphoricum Acidum

Mental weakness leading to physical weakness. Ailments from disappointed love.

Case history

45-year-old man. Presents with a diagnosis of 'chronic fatigue syndrome' with profound physical and mental exhaustion. The illness began with a severe bout of gastroenteritis within a month of his wife leaving him to go and live with another man. He now has a new girlfriend and is most distressed that he is so weak that he cannot sustain an erection long enough to have full sexual intercourse.

Treatment: Phosphoricum Acidum 30c, three times in 24 hours.

Infant snuffles

Sambucus Nigra

Infant snuffles preventing breathing while nursing. Perspiration is the great keynote of this remedy.

Pulsatilla

Yellow mucus, profuse in morning, > open air.

Case history

28-day-old baby with very snuffly breathing which is interfering with breast feeding. Mum particularly remarks on his sweaty head.

Treatment: Sambucus Nigra granules 30c, one pinch on the tongue before last feed of the day.

Infertility

Borax

Galactorrhoea. Menses too soon, profuse, with nausea and stomach pain radiating to small of back.

Natrum Muriaticum

Dryness and burning, smarting in vagina during coition due to dryness.
Premenstrual irritability. < consolation.

Sepia

Bearing down pains, as if uterus would come out – must cross legs.
Apathetic, worn out, can't be bothered with anything.

Case history

29-year-old woman. Married for 4 years. She and her husband have been trying unsuccessfully for a pregnancy since they got married. Has had standard investigations with no abnormal findings. Suffers from premenstrual syndrome in the form of being sad, irritable and exhausted for 10 days before menses. Just wants to be left alone at that time. Doesn't want the husband to be anywhere near her then. Also has dysmenorrhoea with a dragging discomfort in her lower belly.

Treatment: Sepia 10M, three powders over 24 hours.

Influenza

Gelsemium

Slow onset. Thirstless. Heavy limbs (feeling of paralysis). Drowsy. Dull headache > profuse urination.

Mercurius

Profuse sweat. Intolerant of extremes of heat. 'Mapped' tongue (dental imprints). Metallic taste in mouth.

Influenzinum

Single dose after influenza when patient complains of being 'never well since' influenza.

Case history

Local influenza epidemic. House visit to a 30-year-old man with fever, headache, sore, aching, heavy legs and arms. Symptoms have developed over last 48 hours. Can't think. Exhausted. States that his headache is a little better for a while after he urinates. Wife is concerned that he isn't drinking enough fluids.

Treatment: Gelsemium 30c, every 4 hours, as required.

Injuries

Arnica

Bruising injuries. Head injury.

Hypericum

Crush injuries to nerve-rich areas, e.g. fingertips.

Ruta Graveolens

Tendon and ligament injuries and sprains

Ledum

Puncture wounds > cold.

Case history

15-year-old boy. Caught the tip of his right middle finger in the car door. Crush injury without any bony damage.

Treatment: Hypericum 6c, one tablet every 15 minutes or so until pain subsides.

Intermittent
claudication

Cactus
Grandiflorus
Arnica
Camphora

Intermittent claudication

Cactus Grandiflorus

Pain as from constriction by an iron band or tight cord.

Arnica

'Bruised', aching feeling – can't bear to be touched.

Camphora

Icy coldness with cramps in the calves.

Case history

70-year-old man. Has to stop walking every 100 yards with cramping pain in his calves. Absent dorsalis pedis pulse on left. Both popliteal pulses and femoral pulses intact.

Treatment: Cactus Grandiflorus 6c, one tablet sucked at beginning of walking and repeated as often as required. This has allowed him to walk all the way to the local shop and pub 500 yards from his house without stopping.

Mastalgia

Conium

Stony hard breasts. Breasts swollen and painful before and during menses.

Bellis Perennis

Breasts and uterus engorged. Breast pain or pathology especially after injury to breasts.

Phytolacca

Breasts hard and very sensitive. Pain from nipple spreading over whole body.

Case history

30-year-old woman with swollen painful breasts for 14 days before every period. Sore and hard to touch. Loss of sexual desire.

Treatment: Conium 30c, one dose on day 14 of every cycle. Repeat dose every day of discomfort if required.

Measles

Pulsatilla

Profuse, yellow, bland discharges. Conjunctivitis. Worse in warm, stuffy rooms, > open air.

Euphrasia

Profuse, hot, acrid tears < open air.

Sulphur

Burning, itching redness of lids. Hot. Itchy eruptions.

Case history

3-year-old girl. Blonde. Shy. Typical measles rash with a fever over last 4 days. Sore, inflamed eyes, with discharge.

Treatment: Pulsatilla 30c, one tablet three times daily until symptoms improve.

Mumps

Aconite

Sudden onset, especially after exposure to cold wind. Early stages of inflammation.

Mercurius

Profuse sweat. Intolerant of extremes of heat. 'Mapped' tongue (dental imprints). Metallic taste in mouth.

Pulsatilla

Chilly but > open air. Dislikes stuffy rooms. Symptoms constantly changing.

Case history

6-year-old boy during local mumps epidemic. Woke up with fullblown symptoms. Swollen parotid glands and beginning of a fever. Agitated and restless.

Treatment: Aconite 30c, three doses over 24 hours.

Nightmares/night terrors

Belladonna

Sudden. Agitated. Flushed. Hallucinating.

Carcinosin

Waking screaming or shrieking or shrieking during sleep. Familiar things seem strange.

Sulphur

Waking at night with nightmares. Hot. Sticks feet out of bed at night because of heat. Untidy and averse to bathing.

Case history

6-year-old boy. Night terrors since being bitten by a dog. Wakes screaming and afraid with dreams of a big black dog.

Treatment: Belladonna 30c at night until nightmares cease.

Premenstrual syndrome

Lachesis

Violent anger – throws things at people. Jealous. Territorial – drives people away.

Bloated feeling. Can't bear tight things around body or, especially, neck.

Sepia

Worn out. Can't be bothered. Averse to loved ones. Irritable and weary.

Pulsatilla

Great changeability of symptoms. Weepy.
> consolation. Wants company

Case history

32-year-old woman. Violent outbursts of temper before periods. Throws objects in anger at husband. Really wants to hurt him. Drives him out of the house with rage. Abdominal bloating and breast swelling also before period. Symptoms improve immediately at onset of the menstrual flow.

Treatment: Lachesis 200c, one tablet on day 14 of cycle. Repeat dose if symptoms appear.

Recurrent
catarrhal
complaints

Pulsatilla
Kali Bichromum
Hydrastis

Recurrent catarrhal complaints

Pulsatilla

Profuse, bland discharges > open air, < stuffy rooms.
Deafness after a cold.

Kali Bichromum

Stringy, viscid discharges. > heat; < cold.

Hydrastis

Thick, ropy discharges. Eustachian catarrh.

Teething problems

Chamomilla

Frantic, angry, whining.
Wants to be carried and is better when carried.

Calcarea Phosphorica

Thin child with chronic swollen glands.

Merc Sol

Much salivation. Sweaty.

Teething
problems

Chamomilla
Calcarea
Phosphorica
Merc Sol

Case history

14-month-old child. Whining, cross and irritable. Wants to be carried around. One bright red, hot cheek. Teething.

Treatment: Chamomilla 30c granules, one pinch on the tongue every 15 minutes as required.

Tinnitus

China Officinalis

Ringing in the ears associated with fluid loss, e.g. blood or perspiration. Patient may be weak or debilitated from fluid loss.

Graphites

Ringing in ears. Timidity. Weeping with music. < cold weather and around menses.

Spigelia

Noises in ear. Left-sided headache. < tobacco smoke.

HOMEOPATHY IN PRIMARY CARE

Urethral syndrome

Cantharis

Burning, cutting pain in urethra. Urging and/or tenesmus. Increased sexual desire.

Pulsatilla

Symptoms changeable. > gentle motion

Sepia

Bearing down sensation in pelvis – must cross legs. Depressed and irritable. Averse to loved ones.

Case history

45-year-old woman. Six episodes of 'cystitis' in last 12 months. Bacteriology consistently negative. Symptoms are of urging to pass urine and then burning pain in the urethra during micturition.

Treatment: Cantharis 30c, three doses over 24 hours at presentation. Repeat regime at onset of any future symptoms.

Warts

Thuja Occidentalis

Probably the first-line treatment for warts. Can be given either orally as a single dose or applied locally as a mother tincture. Some practitioners combine both approaches.

Causticum

Warts mainly on hands and face. Usually multiple. Large and bleed easily.

Nitricum Acidum

Painful or itchy 'cauliflower' warts which bleed easily.

Unsafe Situation for Allopathic Treatment

Anticipatory anxiety

Argentum Nitricum

Churning in the abdomen. Diarrhoea.
Craves sweets.

Gelsemium

Stage fright. Paralysis – can't go on.
Mind dull and confused.

Lycopodium

Need to be in control. Anxious before event, e.g. public speaking,
then performs well once started.

Anticipatory
anxiety

**Argentum
Nitricum**
Gelsemium
Lycopodium

Childhood problems

See in particular the remedies for infant colic, teething, catarrhal complaints, measles, mumps, etc. Also constitutional remedies are particularly helpful with hyperactivity and problems of sleep disturbance.

Rhus Toxicodendron is often useful for restless boys with enuresis.

Homeopathic remedies are safe to use with all ages of children and for many of these conditions there will be no effective allopathic, safe alternatives.

Dysfunctional labour

Dysfunctional
labour

Caulophyllum
Gelsemium
Cimicifuga
Racemosa

Caulophyllum

Pains fly everywhere – short, painful and ineffectual.

Gelsemium

Anticipation anxiety. Feeling of physical weakness and heaviness, especially of lower limbs.

Cimicifuga Racemosa

Ineffectual pains with depression, gloominess and oversensitivity due to exhaustion.
Pains < least noise.

Case history

22-year-old woman with long first stage in first pregnancy. The contractions are painful but there is slow cervical dilation.

Treatment: Caulophyllum 30c, repeated every 30 minutes until regular, effective contractions are established.

Morning
sickness in
pregnancy

Ipecac
Sepia
Nux Vomica

Morning sickness in pregnancy

Ipecac

Unrelenting vomiting. Nothing helps – no better after vomiting, lying down, etc.

Sepia

Nausea < smell of food.
< putting hands in water, e.g. doing the washing up.

Nux Vomica

Irritable. Fastidious.
Nausea > after vomiting.
Sensation of a stone in the abdomen.

Case history

22-year-old woman. First pregnancy. 10 weeks pregnant.
Incessant nausea and vomiting without relief. Has already had
5 days inpatient treatment with i.v. fluids.

Treatment: Ipecac 30c as often as required.

Problems in the elderly

See the remedies for problems such as diarrhoea, constipation, osteoarthritis, intermittent claudication, night cramps, etc. The major benefit of homeopathy in this group of people is the safety of the remedies.

UNACCEPTABLE SIDE-EFFECT PROFILE

Apart from the treatment of pregnant women, the elderly and infants, unacceptable side-effects tend to be seen mainly with long-term medication. Long-term medication is used, obviously, for chronic conditions, so individualized remedies based on totality are the most useful ones in helping to reduce the need for long-term medication and therefore deal with the problem of unacceptable side-effects, e.g. the problem of NSAIDs in the treatment of arthritic conditions.

The audit work from the Glasgow Homoeopathic Hospital demonstrated a significant number of patients achieving sustained reductions in allopathic treatment after homeopathic care.

Anxiety

Arsenicum Album

Anxiety about health.
Worrier. Fastidious.

Calcarea Carbonica

Lots of fears – in particular, fear of insanity and fear of poverty.
Slow.

Natrum Muriaticum

Anxiety worse in closed spaces and in crowds. Wringing of hands.
< consolation.

Anxiety

Arsenicum Album
Calcarea
Carbonica
Natrum
Muriaticum

Case history

28-year-old male sales executive. Visits the doctor at least
once a month with some concern about a minor symptom. He
is a very hard worker who achieves high standards and is very
particular about his work. Extremely tidy. Makes lists of things to
do almost all the time. Describes himself as a worrier. His tidiness
extends to lining up the cereal boxes 'correctly' on the shelves
whilst shopping at the local supermarket!

Treatment: Arsenicum Album 10M, three doses over 24 hours.

Depression

Calcarea
Carbonica
Sepia
Aurum
Metallicum

Depression

Calcarea Carbonica

Slow. Sluggish. Low energy.
Lots of fears and phobias.

Sepia

Irritable and 'browned off'. Weary. 'Can't be bothered'.
Averse to loved ones.

Aurum Metallicum

Black despondency, hopelessness. Suicidal.

Night cramps

Cuprum Metallicum

Severe, violent, sudden cramps in the calves at night. Cold feet.

Arnica

Cramps in muscles at night after overuse of the muscles, e.g. after significant exertion.

Veratrum Album

Night cramps occurring during a diarrhoeal illness.

Osteoarthritis

Rhus Toxicodendron

< first movement. > motion.
< cold, damp weather.

Bryonia

> rest. < motion.

Causticum

Tearing pains around the joints. Contractions.
> damp, wet weather.

Case history

58-year-old woman. Pain and stiffness in her knees and hands when waking in the morning. The first movements are painful but then the pain eases off. Can't sit for too long without pain getting worse. Knows when it is going to rain because her joints get worse at that time.

Treatment: Rhus Toxicodendron 30c, twice daily for pain and stiffness as required.

REDUCTION OF ALLOPATHIC TREATMENT

Asthma

Arsenicum Album

Anxious. Restless. Asthma worse midnight to 2 a.m. Chilly. Thirst for small quantities frequently.

Kali Carbonicum

Sweating. Weakness. Sharp, cutting, stabbing pains. > sitting forward. Starts at noise.

Natrum Sulphuricum

Worse every change of dry to damp weather. Asthma in children. Worse 4–5 a.m. Must hold chest on coughing.

Asthma

Arsenicum
Album
Kali Carbonicum
Natrum
Sulphuricum

Constipation

Opium

Absolute constipation with no desire. Inactive bowel. After operation. In terminal care, due to opiates.

Silica

Bashful stool – the stool recedes. Painful. Fissure-in-ani.

Calcarea Carbonica

Feels better constipated. Obese. Chilly. Flatulent. Slow in thoughts, habits and action.

Convulsions

Belladonna

Febrile convulsions with fever, red face, dilated pupils and dry mouth. Hallucinations. Restless.

Cuprum Metallicum

Icy cold body. Violent convulsions. Shrieks. Convulsions begin in fingers or toes and spread over whole body.

Plumbum Metallicum

Convulsions with marked aura. Convulsions during menses. Tremors followed by paralysis. < room full of people.

Dysmenorrhoea

Magnesia Phosphorica

Severe cutting pain. Must bend over. > local heat. > pressure.

Colocynthis

Severe pain. > pressure. Angry or suppressed anger. Colicky in nature.

Sepia

Cramping low abdominal discomfort. Bearing down feeling. Must cross legs. Wants to be left alone.

Eczema

Sulphur

Itchy. Hot. Sticks hot feet out of the bed at night. Red orifices. Excoriations. Untidy.

Petroleum

Painful cracks, especially in fingertips. Worse for cold and, therefore, worse in winter. People who handle oil or petrochemical products.

Arsenicum Album

Restless. Chilly. Fastidious. Anxious. Burning pains > hot applications.

Migraine

Natrum Muriaticum

Recurrent hammering headache with visual disturbances. < sunlight. Must wear a hat in the sun. Irritable. Averse to consolation.

Glonione

Bursting, pounding headache. Confusion. Disorientation. Time passes too slowly.

Sanguinaria

Right sided. Sick headache. Settles over the right eye. Begins in the morning and settles by evening. > lying down. > sleep.

Neuralgias

Hypericum

After injuries, especially crush injuries to nerve-rich areas. After fright. < jar. < motion.

Colocynthis

Severe cramping pain. > pressure. Followed by numbness. < after vexation.

Ranunculus Bulbosus

Stitching pains. < touch. < motion. < wet weather. < thinking of complaints.

Psoriasis

Sulphur

Itchy. Hot. Sticks hot feet out of the bed at night. Red orifices. Excoriations. Untidy. Offensive discharges.

Graphites

Chilly. Obese. Timid. Weepy. Sensitive to music. Cracks and excoriations, especially around the ears. Honey-like oozing and/or scales.

Psorinum

Chilly. Despairing. Despair from itching. Forsaken, hopeless feeling. Dirty skin. Thickened skin. < bathing.

SECTION

4

MATERIA MEDICA
A STRUCTURED APPROACH TO LEARNING

Introduction

The pictures of the remedies can be extremely detailed and include symptoms related to every single organ system in the human body. Some of the original materia medicae stretch to ten volumes in size. It is easy, if you have sufficient funds, to fill an entire bookshelf with books of descriptions of the 'drug' pictures of the available homeopathic remedies. But how do you get these patterns into your head? Just as importantly, how do you keep these patterns in your head?

We tend to remember new facts by using mental 'hooks'. We link the new information to some existing information in our minds or we link the name of the remedy to some striking features of the remedy. These striking features are 'strange, rare and peculiar' symptoms, well-established indications or keynotes.

This section of the book introduces all the remedies in 'List A' of the UK Faculty of Homoeopathy examination requirements. This has been accepted throughout Europe and the United States as a basic list of remedies of which a homeopathic specialist should have a good working knowledge.

It is useful to consider four levels of knowledge in relation to each remedy.

Level 1

A 'notable' symptom. This is a single statement about the remedy. This may be a 'strange, rare or peculiar' symptom which would make the practitioner think of this particular remedy. Alternatively, this symptom may be a 'well established indication' for this remedy.

Level 2

The keynotes (including major modalities). As presented here, homeopathic knowledge at this level includes about five keynotes, plus the most notable ameliorating and aggravating factors. Together these present a succinct collection of 'hooks' on which to base the next level of knowledge. These five keynotes are not necessarily the most important features of the remedy, but are amongst its most distinctive features. If you memorize this information you will have a good starting knowledge of the remedies on which to build.

Level 3

Condensed materia medica – this covers a much wider range of symptoms relating to the whole human body.The main features of the remedy are illustrated. The shorter materia medicae such as Boericke, Phatak and Clarke are good examples of this.

Level 4

In depth study – this includes a description of the source material and its toxicology, a description of the main features of the remedy including its 'essence' and its main themes and cross referencing to other remedies by making comparisons with and studying the relationship to them.

This book includes learning about remedies to a depth of the first two of these four levels. This gives a good grounding and secure 'hooks' on which to base a deeper and wider knowledge by exploring levels 3 and 4 of selected remedies.

You should be aware, however, that some of these remedies are known to have many more uses than others. In fact, remedies which have a wide number of uses, and are therefore commonly indicated, are known as 'polychrests'. However, whether a remedy is, or is not, a 'polychrest', the basic information contained in this section provides a good, fundamental understanding of each remedy.

Example

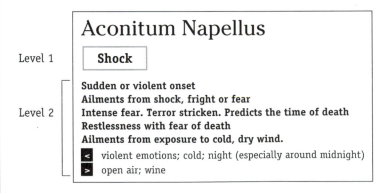

Level 1

Aconitum Napellus

Shock

Level 2

Sudden or violent onset
Ailments from shock, fright or fear
Intense fear. Terror stricken. Predicts the time of death
Restlessness with fear of death
Ailments from exposure to cold, dry wind.

< violent emotions; cold; night (especially around midnight)
> open air; wine

Note: The conventional symbols of < and >, representing 'worse with' and 'better with' respectively, are used throughout this section.

HOMEOPATHY IN PRIMARY CARE

Aconitum Napellus

> **Shock**

Sudden or violent onset
Ailments from shock, fright or fear
Intense fear. Terror stricken. Predicts the time of death
Restlessness with fear of death
Ailments from exposure to cold, dry wind.

< violent emotions; cold; night (especially around midnight)
> open air; wine

Agaricus
Muscarius

Clumsiness and
involuntary,
exaggerated
movements

Agaricus Muscarius

> **Clumsiness and involuntary, exaggerated movements**

Dullness in morning
Involuntary, exaggerated movements – chorea, twitches or cramps
Very sensitive to cold
Stitching, splinter-like pains
Pain in spine, sensitive to pressure and touch

 cold; morning; alcohol; pressure and touch
> evening

Allium Cepa

> **Excoriating nasal discharge with bland lachrymation**

Headache > open air and < returning to warm room
Sneezing < returning to warm room
Catarrhal hoarseness
Cough compels patient to grasp larynx
Dullness of mind

< evening; warm room; dampness
> open air; cold room

Aloe

Sore, tender
haemorrhoids
protrude like
grapes, > cold
water

Aloe

> ## Sore, tender haemorrhoids protrude like grapes, > cold water

Jelly-like mucus from throat and rectum
Hungry, during diarrhoea
Burning, offensive, flatulent rectal discharge relieves abdominal pain
Urge to stool in morning and after eating
Feeling of weakness in anal sphincter

< early morning; hot, dry weather; after eating or drinking
> cold water; cold weather; from discharge of flatus and stool

Alumina

Dryness of body and mind

Craves indigestibles
Constipation
Time passes too slowly
Tottering and falling when closing eyes
**Weak memory, inability to think coherently and confusion of
identity**

< Warmth, warm room; speaking; dry weather; on waking early
> evening; open air; damp weather; cold washing

Ammonium Carbonicum

Livid, weak and drowsy

Heart failure with exertional dyspnoea
Epistaxis when washing in the morning and after eating
Mouth breathing because nose stuffed at night. Infant snuffles
Aversion to washing
Cold. Averse to open air

< damp, cloudy weather; open air; during menses; 3–4 a.m.
> pressure; eating; lying on abdomen

Anacardium

> ## Sensation of a plug or a band

Ill-natured, cursing, malicious
Vacillating. Bad memory
Feeling of having two opposing wills
Itchy skin < scratching
Gastric pain relieved by eating, then worse in 3 hours

< mental exertion; anger, fright; stepping heavily; rubbing
> eating; hot bath

Antimonium Crudum

Tongue coating thick and white

Disordered digestion
Aversion to being looked at and to being touched
Lumps – in watery stool, leucorrhoea, skin, nails
Cracks – nostrils, angles of mouth, canthi
Sentimental mood in moonlight

 cold; cold bathing; heat of summer, overheating; overeating
▶ open air; rest; lying down

Antimonium Tartaricum

Antimonium
Tartaricum

Great accumulation of mucus with rattling

Great
accumulation of
mucus with
rattling

Great weakness, profuse cold clammy sweat and sleepiness
Chronic trembling of head and hands
Coarse, loose, rattling cough
Clings to attendants. Child wants to be carried
Nausea with frequent vomiting of bitter, sour substances

< warm room, wraps, weather; Anger; Lying
> expectoration; sitting erect; motion; vomiting

Apis Mellifica

Puffy tissues

Sudden, stinging, burning pains which make the patient cry out
Bruised soreness, very sensitive to touch
Oedematous swellings without thirst
Difficulty passing urine
Jealous, fussy and fidgety

< hot room; hot drinks; hot bath; touch
> cool air; motion

Argentum Nitricum

Anticipation anxiety with diarrhoea and flatulence

Craves sugar, which aggravates symptoms
Palpitations and tremors
Violent pains, like deeply embedded splinter
Impulsive and hurried
Craves fresh air

< anxiety; sugar
> cool air

Arnica Montana

Bruises

Very painful, bruised soreness
Never well since injury
Fears being struck, touched or approached
Apathetic. Says nothing ails him
Haemorrhagic tendency

< injuries; jarring; touch
> lying with head low or lying outstretched

Arsenicum Album

> ## Sickness and diarrhoea with prostration and restlessness

Chilly
Thirst for small sips frequently
Burning pains, > heat
Restless anxiety
Acrid, scanty, thin discharges

< midnight to 2 a.m.; cold food and drink; exertion
> hot applications; hot food; elevating head

Aurum Metallicum

| Suicidal depression |

Heart disease with violent palpitations
Weak but very sensitive to pain
Offensive breath
Painful nose, sensitive to touch
Hopelessness

< emotions; mental exertion; cold weather; night
> cold bathing; music; walking

Baptisia

> ## Sense of duality. Parts of body feel separated or scattered about

Sense of duality.
Parts of body feel
separated or
scattered about

Rapid prostration

Sore, bruised feeling, aching, heavy muscles

Foul odour of body and secretions

Dusky, sodden, besotted appearance

Dull, confused. Falls asleep while answering question

< mental exertion; swallowing solids; in closed room; humid

> motion; drinking liquids; open air

Baryta Carbonica

Dwarfish, physically and mentally

Slow mentally. Senility
Aversion to strangers
Enlarged, indurated glands, especially tonsils, neck and prostate
Great tendency to take colds
Paralytic effects

< company; cold; lying on painful part
> warm atmosphere; warm coverings

Belladonna

> **Sudden. Red, hot and dry**

Delirium
Throbbing head
Bright red glossy skin
Jerks and spasms
Oversensitiveness of all senses

< draught; light; noise; touch; jarring
> rest; bending backward

Bellis Perennis

> **Deep trauma or septic wounds, especially abdominal**

Sore and bruised feeling in muscles

Nerve injuries > cold bathing

Venous stasis and varicose veins

Fullness about the spleen

Never well since injury

< injuries; sprains; touch; becoming chilled when hot

> continued motion; local cold applications

Berberis Vulgaris

> ## Biliary and urinary calculi

Pains rapidly changing character and locality, radiating out from one point
Cough associated with fistulae in other parts
Backache with severe prostration
Mentally and physically tired
Vaginismus and diminished sexual desire

◀ motion; jarring; stepping hard
▶ after urination

Borax

Aphthous and
catarrhal
conditions with
thick, hot
discharges

Borax

Aphthous and catarrhal conditions with thick, hot discharges

Vertigo going downstairs. Great dread of downward motion
Sensitive to and violent fright from sudden sounds, thunder
Entropion. Blepharitis
Dry skin. Festers easily and heals slowly
Infertility

< downward motion; sudden noises
> 11 p.m.; pressure; holding painful side

Bowel nosodes

The bowel nosodes were prepared from stool cultures. They are used in the treatment of chronic disease and are usually given only once, with no repeat for several months. They are most commonly used when there is no one clear remedy, but strong features of a group of related remedies.

Bacillus No. 7

Mental and physical fatigue

Related to the Kali salts, bromine and iodine.

Dysentery Co.

Nervous tension

Related to Argentum Nitricum, Arsenicum Album, Kalmia, Lycopodium and Nux Vomica.

Gaertner

Malnutrition

Related to Mercurius, Phosphorus and Silica.

Morgan Co.

Congestion

Related to Calcarea Carbonica, Graphites, Petroleum, Psorinum and Sulphur.

Proteus

Suddenness and violence of symptoms

Related to Apis Mellifica, Cuprum Metallicum, Ignatia, Natrum Muriaticum.

Sycotic Co.

Irritation, especially of mucous membranes

Related to Bacillinum, Natrum Sulphuricum, Nitricum Acidum, Thuja Occidentalis.

Bryonia

Stitching or bursting pains < least motion

Dryness of mucous membranes
Thirst for large quantities infrequently
Large, dry, hard stools
Pleurisy
Stony hard, heavy breasts which must be supported – before menses

< motion; touch; heat; eating
> pressure; lying on painful side; cool, open air

Cactus Grandiflorus

Sensations of constrictions

Angina – 'As if an iron hand was around the heart'
Periodicity of symptoms, especially neuralgic pains
Haemorrhage – from nose, lungs, stomach, rectum or bladder
Whole body feels tight or caged
Intermittent claudication

< lying down; at 11 a.m. and 11 p.m.
> open air; rest

Calcarea Carbonica

Overweight, cold, flatulent and sweaty

Glandular swellings
Slow, sluggish
Limp, cold, damp handshake
Craves indigestibles – chalk, etc.
'Just sits'

< cold; physical and mental exertion; pressure of clothes; milk; dentition

> rubbing; lying on back; dark

Calcarea Phosphorica

> ### Headache of schoolchildren with diarrhoea

Craves ham, bacon, salted or smoked meat
Aids formation of callus in fractures
Coldness or soreness in spots
Flabby, sunken abdomen
Thin, brittle bones and swollen glands

< damp; changes in weather; melting snow; dentition; loss of fluids
> summer; lying down

Calcarea Sulphurica

Tendency to suppuration

Abscesses – after lancing and once it is discharging
Skin won't heal. Eczema with yellow scales
Thick, yellow discharges
Rattling mucus in chest
Burning soles

< draughts; during night; cold; wet
> after washing; uncovering; open air

Calendula Officinalis

Injuries causing torn or ragged wounds

Pain excessive and out of all proportion
Prevents formation of sepsis
Sensitive to damp or open air
Easily frightened
Tendency to take colds

< damp weather; cloudy weather; evening
> warmth

Camphora

Icy cold, yet averse to covers

Collapse with cold nose and skin, anxiety and restlessness
Burning in stomach
Anguish and hysteria
Impotence with coldness of sexual organs
Pains disappear when thinking of them

◄ when half asleep; cold; suppressions
► free discharges; sweat; thinking of complaint

Cantharis

Cystitis. Burning, scalding pain when urinating

Terrible urging and tenesmus or dribbling
Retention of urine with cutting pains
Burning, cutting pains in body cavities
Increased sexual desire. Sexual frenzy
Expels placenta, moles, products of conception

< urinating; coffee; sight or sound of water; bright objects
> rubbing; rest

Carbo Vegetalis

Weakness from loss of fluids

Flatulence with colic
Air hunger. Wants to be fanned
Weak, sick, exhausted, cold breath and copious cold sweat
Never well since debilitating illness
Bleeding, spongy gums

◄ morning; on rising; warmth; exhausting diseases; butter, pork or fat food

► Eructations; being fanned; loosening clothing around waist

Carcinosin

Family history of cancer

Fastidious
Love of animals and nature
Likes thunderstorms
Better or worse at the seashore
Desire for butter, chocolate

< seashore; approach of storm; short sleep
> seashore; approach of storm; physical exertion

Caulophyllum

Irregular, weak labour pains

Sharp short, erratic ineffectual pains in early labour
Pains are spasmodic and fly about from one place to another
Fretful and easily displeased, with internal tremor
Exhaustion and spasmodic after-pains after long labour
Painful stiffness in small joints of hands and feet

 pregnancy; during menses; coffee; open air
▶ warmth

Causticum

Urinary incontinence with cough

Morning hoarseness and aphonia
Paralysis of eyelids or face due to exposure to dry, cold winds
Rheumatic disease with contractions and deformities
Soreness and rawness of scalp, throat, respiratory tract, rectum, urethra, vagina, etc.
Ailments from long-lasting grief

< dry, cold winds; after coffee; 3–4 a.m. or evening; extremes of temperature
> damp, wet weather; warmth; cold drink

Chamomilla

Teething infant

Child wants to be carried and is then more quiet
Twitchings and convulsions during teething
Frantic irritability with intolerance of pain
Ugly, cross, uncivil and quarrelsome
Colic after anger

◀ anger; night; dentition; coffee
▶ being carried; warm, wet weather

Chelidonium Majus

Right-sided symptoms. Liver disease

Jaundice. Icterus. Biliary disorders
Liver pains radiating backward
Right lung infection
Pain under right scapula
Right foot cold, left foot warm

< change of weather; motion; 4 a.m. and 4 p.m.
> hot drinks; hot food; bending backward

China Officinalis

Debility from loss of fluids

Profuse, exhausting discharges
Haemorrhages from any body orifice
Lienteric, bloody stools
Drenching sweats at night
Ravenous hunger, especially at night

< alternate days; loss of vital fluids; touch; fruit
> hard pressure; loose clothes

Cimicifuga Racemosa

> **Spasmodic, severe, ineffectual labour pains
> < least noise**

Depressed, gloomy and oversensitive from exhaustion
Trembling and twitching
Headache pressing outward or upward (as if top of head would fly off)
Intense ache in or behind eyeballs
Rheumatic muscular aches shooting or wandering here and there

< menstruation; cold, damp air; alcohol
> warm wraps; gentle continued motion; open air

Cimicifuga
Racemosa

Spasmodic,
severe,
ineffectual
labour pains
< least noise

Cina

Child grinds
teeth and picks
and bores at
nose

> ## Child grinds teeth and picks and bores at nose

Hates to be looked at and touched
Angry, irritable, petulant and dissatisfied
Ravenous hunger. Hungry soon after eating
Twitchings and spasms
Pale, sickly look. Bluish about the mouth

◀ touch; being looked at; during sleep
▶ lying on abdomen

Cocculus

Travel sickness

Nausea with giddiness
Empty hollow feeling
Aversion to food when merely looking at it
One-sided paralysis and paralysis of single parts
Takes everything in bad part. Time passes too quickly

< motion of boats and cars; loss of sleep
> lying quietly in a warm room

Coffea Cruda

Nervous sleeplessness

Overexcitable; oversensitive; overacute
Mind full of ideas and therefore wakeful
Hearing acute. Wakes at least sound
Skin painfully sensitive
Toothache relieved by ice water

< noise; mental exertion; emotions
> sleep; lying; warmth

Colocynthis

Colic

Severe sudden cramping pain > firm pressure
Paroxysmal, sharp, spasmodic right-sided sciatica
Neuralgic pains > pressure, followed by numbness
Watery diarrhoea worse after eating or drinking
Frequent urge to urinate. Scanty amounts of urine

< emotions; vexation; lying on painless side
> hard pressure; heat; gentle motion

Conium

Stony hard indurations in breasts

Hard sore glands
Great sensitivity to light without inflammation of eyes
Vertigo < least motion of eyes or head
Hot flushes or sweat on falling asleep
Stopping and starting of urinary flow

< seeing moving objects; alcohol
> letting affected part hang down

Crataegus

Heart failure

Dyspnoea on exertion
Cardiac dilation
Weak and exhausted
Insomnia
Apprehensive, irritable and despondent

< warm room; least exertion; night
> fresh air; rest; quiet

Cuprum Metallicum

Cramps

Spasmodic violent cramps and convulsions
Illnesses from non-appearance or suppression of eruptions or
discharges
Icy cold body
Cough relieved by drink of cold water
Vomiting relieved by cold water

< suppressions; hot weather; touch
> cold drinks; pressure

Drosera

Cough

Incessant or spasmodic barking or choking cough
Whooping cough with epistaxis
Cough beginning as soon as head hits the pillow at night
Sensation of a feather in the larynx
Aversion to pork

< lying down; after midnight; talking
> open air; pressure

Dulcamara

> ## Catarrhal, rheumatic and urticarial problems
> ## < cold and damp

Confused. Speech difficult
Cutting pain around umbilicus followed by green, slimy stools
Exanthema like nettle rash
Rheumatic symptoms alternating with diarrhoea or eruptions
Ailments from exposure to constant changes of temperature

< cold, wet; being chilled while hot; suppressed eruptions
> motion; warmth; dry weather

Eupatorium Perfoliatum

Violent, aching, bone-breaking pains

Very restless. Can't keep still despite great desire to do so
Not relieved by motion
Intermittent fever with chill commencing about 7–9 a.m.
Vomits water, food or bile as the chill passes off
Insatiable thirst before and during chill

- **<** cold air; periodically; motion
- **>** vomiting bile; sweating; lying on face

Euphrasia

> **Profuse, acrid lachrymation with profuse, bland coryza**

Aversion to light
Daytime only cough with excessive lachrymation
After trauma to eye
Painful menses lasting only an hour or a day
Amenorrhoea with ophthalmia

< sunlight; wind; warmth
> open air; winking; wiping eyes

Ferrum Metallicum

> ## Red parts become white – lips, face, tongue

Red parts become
white – lips, face,
tongue

Changeable mood
Restlessness, driving out of bed
Oversensitiveness
Aversion to drinking during headache
Obesity

< night; emotions; anger; violent exertion; eating; sweats
> gentle motion

Ferrum
Phosphor-
icum

Early stages of
febrile illness,
before exudation
sets in

Ferrum Phosphoricum

Early stages of febrile illness, before exudation sets in

Full, soft, flowing pulse
Venous congestion with haemorrhages and blood-streaked discharges
Soreness and bleeding after operation
Aversion to milk and meat. Vomiting of undigested food
Menses every 3 weeks with bearing down sensation

< night; 4–6 a.m.; checked sweat; noise
> cold applications; bleedings; lying down

Gelsemium

Stage fright

Anticipatory anxiety. Paralysis
Aching, heavy weakness and soreness of limbs, e.g. influenza
Slow onset
Headache preceded by blindness or > passing urine
Thirstless

< damp weather; emotions; dread
> profuse urination; sweating; alcoholic drinks

Glonione

Bursting, pounding headache

Violent palpitations
Indicated in high blood pressure in aged
Confusion. Disoriented in place
Time passes too slowly
Sensation of pulsation throughout body. Pulsating pains

 heat on head; heat of sun; hot weather; motion; jar; shaking; injury; suppressed menses; cutting hair

> open air; elevating head; cold things

Graphites

Graphites

Thickened, scaly or crusty patches on skin

Thickened, scaly or crusty patches on skin

Flatulence. Dyspepsia > temporarily from eating
Skin eruptions with oozing, sticky exudates
Anxiety in morning on waking
Inclination to sit
Weeping from music

< cold; light; during and after menses
> open air; eating; touch

Hamamelis Virginica

| Hard, knotty, swollen varicose veins |

Haemorrhoids. Protruding, with raw feeling in anus
Bruised soreness of affected parts
Epistaxis
Haemoptysis, with scarcely any effort
Metrorrhagia

< injuries; pressure; open air
> rest; lying quietly

Hepar Sulphuris Calcareum

Pus. Suppuration

Hurried. Dissatisfied. Disposition to contradict
Violent rage leading to violent deeds
Chilly
Sweats easily
Oversensitive to all impressions. Sticking, sore pains

< cold, dry air; cold wind; draughts; least uncoveirng; touch
> heat; damp weather; warm wraps

Hydrastis

> **Breast cancer. Hard, adherent. Peau d'orange. Nipple retracted**

Thick, ropy discharges – nose, vagina, bladder
Flabby, large tongue showing imprints of teeth
Eustachian catarrh
Irritability after dinner. Malicious
Broken down by excessive use of alcohol

< cold air; inhaling air; old age
> pressure; warm covering

Hypericum

> ## Injuries to nerves or nerve-rich areas

Crush injuries to fingers
Punctured or penetrating wounds. Lacerations
Complaints from fright
Mistakes in writing or speaking
Asthma after spinal injury

- **<** injury; jar; shock; motion
- **>** lying on face; bending backward

Ignatia

Ailments from disappointed love and silent grief

Sighing
Incredible changeability of mood. Laughter to sadness and tears
Sensation of a lump
**Contradictoriness of symptoms, e.g. sore throat > swallowing;
piles > walking; empty stomach, not > eating**
Consolation and conversation <

< grief; worry; touch; coffee; tobacco
> swallowing; eating; lying on affected part

Iodum

Goitre and hyperthyroidism

Always too hot
Anxious, cross and restless
Aversion to people
Ravenous hunger, yet loses weight
Croup caused by long-continued damp weather

< heat
> cold; air; bathing

Ipecacuanha

Continuous nausea unrelieved by vomiting

Violent, spasmodic cough causing vomiting

Rattling in chest without expectoration

Face – one side hot, other side cold

Anxiety during fever

Bright red menstrual haemorrhage with nausea

< warmth; damp; overeating

> open air

Kali Bichromium

Pains migrate quickly from place to place

Stringy, viscid discharges – nose, saliva, eyes, ears, chest, vagina
Infant snuffles in fat, chubby babies
Pains in small spots (can be covered by one finger)
Ulcers
Indifferent and apathetic

< cold; damp; morning; undressing
> heat; motion

Kali Carbonicum

Sweat, backache and weakness

Sharp, cutting, stabbing pains
Weakness of muscles, heart, intellect
Intolerance of cold and cold weather
Starts from noise. Shrieks at trifles
Swelling of eyelids

◄ cold; air; winter; lying on painful side
► warmth; sitting bent

Kali Phosphoricum

> **Want of nerve power. Mental and physical depression**

Putrid secretions and odour
Irritability and nervous dread. < mental exertion
Oversensitivity
Dry mouth. Halitosis
Nervous 'gone' feeling in stomach. Hungry soon after eating

< worry; mental and physical exertion
> sleep; eating; gentle motion

Kali
Phosphor-
icum

Want of nerve
power. Mental
and physical
depression

Kali Sulphuricum

Profuse, deep yellow discharges

Hurried. Anger. Anxiety > open air
Psoriasis. Desquamation. Yellow scales
Yellow watery discharges from skin ulcers
Desires sweets, cold food and drink
Rattling mucus in chest

< warmth; consolation; noise
> cold air; walking; fasting

Kreosotum

> **Acrid, hot, foul discharges, especially genitourinary**

Colicky pains during and especially after menses
Restlessness at night
Sensitive to or weeping from music
Painful dentition. Rapid decay of teeth and spongy, bleeding gums
Urinary urging with offensive urine. Urinary incontinence while lying

- **<** dentition; cold; rest; eating; lying; 6 p.m. to 6 a.m.
- **>** warmth; hot food; motion; pressure; after sleep

Lac Caninum

Sore throat. Alternating sides

All pains right to left and back again
Very forgetful. Makes purchases and walks away without them
Delusions of snakes and spiders
Desire for company. Fear of fainting
Galactorrhoea. Helps to dry up breast milk

< touch; jar; during menses; cold air
> cold drinks; open air

HOMEOPATHY IN PRIMARY CARE

Lachesis

> ### Jealousy

Cannot bear tight clothing, especially around neck
Haemorrhages. All symptoms > flow
Loquacity
Flushes of heat
Wants to be fanned, but at a distance and slowly

- ◀ sleep; after sleep; morning; heat, of summer, of spring, of sun; empty swallowing; swallowing liquids; pressure; pressure of clothes; alcohol
- ▶ open air; free discharges; flow; cold drinks; loosening clothes

Ledum

Puncture wounds > cold applications

Lack of vital heat
Pain in small joints
Angry. Dissatisfied. Aversion to people
Anal fissures
Insect bites and stings which burn

< warmth; injury; motion of joints
> cold; bathing

HOMEOPATHY IN PRIMARY CARE

Lilium Tigrinum

Lilium
Tigrinum

Acts mainly on
venous
circulation and
female organs

> **Acts mainly on venous circulation and female organs**

Full, heavy or forced out feeling
Hurried. Desires to do several things at once
Consolation <
Menses flow only when moving about
Palpitation during pregnancy

< warmth; miscarriage; consolation
> cool, open, fresh air; when busy; crossing legs

Lycopodium

Flatulent dyspepsia

Symptoms left to right
Full of gas. Acidity
Apprehensive about new things
Love of power. Desire to be in control
Lack of confidence

< 4–8 p.m.; warmth; pressure of clothes; eating
> warm drinks; motion; urinating; belching

HOMEOPATHY IN PRIMARY CARE

Magnesia Phosphorica

> **Dysmenorrhoea > local heat**

Cramps, convulsions, neuralgic pains
Complains all the time about the pain
Toothache > heat and hot drinks
Thirst for very cold drinks
Colic, making patient bend double

< cold; air; night; milk
> warmth; hot bathing; rubbing; pressure; bending double

Medorrhinum

Asthma > lying on face and protruding tongue

Hurried. Time passes too slowly
> Evening. Night people
Shuns responsibilities. Biting nails
History of early heart disease in parents
Breasts and nipples sore and sensitive to touch

 damp; daytime; 3–4 a.m.; thunderstorm

> lying on abdomen; hard rubbing; fresh air; damp weather; seashore

Mercurius (Merc Sol)

Mercurius

Can't tolerate
extremes of heat
or cold

> ## Can't tolerate extremes of heat or cold

Sweating profuse
Salivation profuse
Metallic taste in mouth. Teeth-indented tongue
Ulcerations
Bloody, slimy stool < at night

< night;,sweating; lying on right side; when heated; draughts;
damp cold

> moderate temperature; rest

Mercurius Corrosivus

Tenesmus of rectum, not > stool

Internal burnings and constrictions
Anxious and restless. Rocks fast
Dysphagia on attempting to swallow a drop of liquid
Urine passed drop by drop with intense burning
Continuous urge to stool. 'Never get done' feeling

< after urination and stool; swallowing; night; cold
> rest; warm application

Mezereum

Shingles

Painful eruptions sensitive to cold
Obstinate twitching of left upper eyelid
Craves ham, fat, coffee, wine
Intolerable itching
Eruptions ulcerate, from thick scabs with pus underneath

< night; suppressions; warmth
> wrapping up; eating; open air

Natrum Carbonicum

Reserved. Unselfish. Tendency to sacrifice

Very nervous during thunderstorm
Weak digestion with sour belching
Hungry at 5 a.m.
Headache from mental exertion or sunlight
Thick, foul, yellow or green nasal discharge

< heat; sun; 5 a.m.; mental or physical exertion
> eating; pressing; rubbing

Natrum Muriaticum

Ailments from grief

Consolation <
Irritable. Bears grudges. Can't cry
Headaches and migraines < sunlight
Desires salt. Aversion to bread, slimy food
Greasy skin with flexural eczema

< sun; heat; exertion; consolation; puberty
> open air; sweating

Natrum Phosphoricum

Sourness

Fearful. Starting easily. Starts at noise
Blisters on tip of tongue
Dysphagia
Sour belching, sour vomiting and greenish diarrhoea
Trembling feeling

◀ sugar; thunderstorms
▶ cold

Natrum Sulphuricum

Mental ill effects of head injury

Averse to life. Suicidal thoughts of shooting or hanging
Desire for salty fish, beer and cold drinks
Flatulence
Worse every change of dry to damp weather
Asthma in children, dampness, 4–5 a.m. Must hold chest on
coughing

< damp; head injury; late evening; lying on left side
> open air; warm dry air; change of position

Nitricum Acidum

Pains sticking like splinters

Offensive discharges
Anxiety about health
Hatred of persons who had offended
Oversensitive, especially to noise
Craves fat, herring, salt

< touch; jar; cold; noise; damp; night
> riding in a carriage; gliding motion

Nux Vomica

Anger and digestive disturbances

Fastidious. Angry and impatient
Hard-working, hard-living person. Craves stimulants
Nausea > after vomiting. Feeling like a stone in the stomach
Vertigo, especially with momentary loss of consciousness
Headache in the morning or in sunshine

- **<** early morning; cold; open air; uncovering; high living; slight causes
- **>** free discharges; wrapping head; milk

Opium

> ## Obstinate constipation, especially from use of opiates

Sleepy. Somnambulism
Indifference to pleasure or suffering
Paralyses – of bowel, extremities
Twitching, numbness and jerks
Retention of urine after confinement

◄ emotions; fear; alcohol; suppressed discharges
► cold; uncovering; coffee

Petroleum

Cracking eczema in cold weather

Rough, hard, thickened and fissured skin
Motion sickness
Nausea and waterbrash, especially in morning
Diarrhoea only in daytime
Confusion of mind while walking

< motion; winter; cold; dampness;
> warm dry air

Phosphoricum Acidum

Mental, then physical, weakness

Apathetic. Wants nothing and cares for nothing
Ailments from disappointed love and silent grief
Pains in back of head from exhausted nerve power or excessive grief
Diarrhoea. Profuse, painless, dirty white or lienteric
Frequent urination of copious amounts

 loss of fluids; fatigue; emotions; sexual excess; cold; draughts
> warmth; short sleep

Phosphorus

> ## Sympathetic and very sensitive to others' upset

Fears – something will happen; imaginary things; insanity; dark; thunderstorms
Haemorrhages
Averse to warm food and drink
Thirst for cold drinks which are vomited once the water turns warm
Desires ice cream; salt; cheese; chocolate

< lying on left side; emotions; cold; putting hands in cold water; warm food

> eating; sleep

Phytolacca

Burning hot sore
throat. Cannot
even swallow
water

Phytolacca

> **Burning hot sore throat. Cannot even swallow water**

Pain in throat shoots to ears
Mumps
Rheumatism of fibrous tissues
Sore, aching, bruised feeling over whole body < movement
Mastitis. Hard and sensitive. Pain spreads over whole body

◄ damp; hot drinks; motion; rising from bed
► lying on abdomen or left side; rest; dry weather

Platinum

Haughty. Arrogant. Contemptuous

Sadness > open air
Local coldness and numbness
Violent, cramping, numbing pains followed by spasms
Will almost go into spasm from vaginal examination
Will almost faint during coition

< emotions; coition; touch; nerve exhaustion
> walking in open air

Plumbum Metallicum

Progressive paralyses and contractions

Extensors of upper limbs mainly affected
Sharp, lightning-like, neuralgic pains hips to knees
Depression. Unable to find proper words when talking
Colic. Abdomen feels drawn inwards
Constipation. Hard, black stools. Anus feels painfully contracted

< exertion; clear weather; company; room full of people
> hard pressure; rubbing; stretching limbs

Podophyllum

> ## Profuse, gushing, painless diarrhoea, preceded by gurgling

Loquacity and whining
Teeth grinding. Burning sensation of tongue
Thirst for large quantities of cold water
Diarrhoea during teething with hot, glowing cheeks
Vaginal prolapse, especially after childbirth

- **<** early morning; eating; hot weather
- **>** rubbing or stroking liver; lying on abdomen

Psorinum

Itchy skin conditions

Offensive discharges
Recurrent ailments
Anxiety. Despair from itching. Forsaken feeling
Inflamed orifices with foul discharges
Stool dark, brown, gushing. Penetrating odour

< cold; washing; changing weather; stormy weather; suppressions
> lying with head low; profuse sweating; hard pressure

Pulsatilla

Changeability of symptoms

Timid. Weepy. > company
Chilly but > open air. Dislikes stuffy rooms
Thirstless. Averse to fat
> gentle motion
Catarrhal complaints. Styes and conjunctivitis

< warmth; rest; beginning of motion; rich foods; fat
> cold; open air; after crying; lying on back

Pyrogenium

Septic fevers

All discharges horribly offensive
Bruised, sore, aching feeling with prostration
Septic puerperal fever
Pulse and temperature out of proportion
Aching in all limbs and bones. Bed feels too hard

< cold, damp; motion; moving eyes
> heat; hot bath; changing position

Ranunculus Bulbosus

> **Painful, bruised chest < touch, motion and in wet, stormy weather**

Pleurodynia, pleurisy or shingles. Stitching pains
Bad effects of alcohol. Delirium tremens
< thinking of complaints
Crawling and tingling feeling in fingers
Eruptions – burning and intense itching. Bluish vesicles

< air; cold; damp; motion; change of temperature; change of position

> warm application; warm weather; standing; rest

Ranunculus
Bulbosus

Painful, bruised
chest < touch,
motion and in
wet, stormy
weather

Rhus
Toxicoden-
dron

Joint pains
< 1st movement;
> motion; < rest

Rhus Toxicodendron

Joint pains < 1st movement; > motion; < rest

Pain and stiffness < damp weather
Irritability and restlessness at night, driving out of bed
Back pains and stiffness compelling constant movement in bed
Urticaria, vesicles. Least cold air makes skin painful
Asthma alternating with skin eruptions

 exposure to wet; cold; before storms; rest; 1st movement
heat; continued motion; rubbing; hot bath

Rumex Crispus

Rumex
Crispus

Many varied
pains, neither
fixed nor
constant
anywhere

> **Many varied pains, neither fixed nor constant anywhere**

**Cough from tickling in throat. Every breath of cold air <
Sticky secretions from mucous membranes with burning
Intense itch, especially lower limbs < cold air when undressing
Meat causes belching and pruritus**

- **<** cold air; inhaling; changes of temperature
- **>** covering mouth; wrapping up

Ruta Graveolens

Tendon injuries

**Bruised, sore, aching and restless. Especially affects flexor
tendons**
Eyestrain
Violent thirst for ice-cold water
Difficult stool with rectal prolapse
Lower limbs heavy

< cold; damp; lying; sitting; eyestrain
> warmth; lying on back

Sabadilla

> ## Violent sneezing with itching in nose

Lachrymation on going into open air
Sore throat, left to right, < empty swallowing
Weakness, nervousness and startling. Formication
Imagine they have very serious disease, e.g. cancer
Thirstless. Desire for hot things

< cold; periodically
> open air; heat

Sabina

Threatened miscarriage about 3rd month

Music intolerable – 'goes through the bone and marrow'
Gout. Red, shiny swelling of small joints
Desire for lemonade, lemons
Pain from sacrum to pubis
Menses profuse, bright

< heat; night; foggy weather; pregnancy; climacteric
> cold

Sambucus Nigra

Infant snuffles

Profuse perspiration
Constant fretfulness
Anxiety at night and on waking
Paroxysmal, suffocative cough coming on about midnight
Dry, burning heat at night with profuse sweat without thirst
during waking hours

< dry, cold air; midnight; fruit
> motion; sitting up in bed

Sanguinaria

Migraine

Right-sided, sick headache, settles over right eye
Hot flushes at climacteric. Burning redness of cheeks, palms and soles
Burning sensation in eyes and ears
Pain over liver. Vomiting bile. Jaundice
Nasal polyps. Coryza followed by diarrhoea

< sun; light; odours; jar; periodically; climacteric
> sleep; lying on back; vomiting

Secale Cornutum

> **Irregular heavy menses**

Great sense of heat through whole body
All symptoms > cold
Debility, anxiety, emaciation though appetite and thirst may be excessive
Twitchings, spasms and cramps
Discharges dark, thin, foul and exhausting

◄ warmth; just before and during menses; covers
► cold; bathing; forcible stretching

Sepia

'Brown and down'

Depressed and irritable. Anger from contradiction
Aversion to loved ones
'Can't be bothered'. Weeping < consolation
Bearing down pains – must cross legs
Desires vinegar, pickles and acids. Aversion to fats

◀ cold; air; before menses; 4–6 p.m.
▶ dancing; violent exercise; warmth

Silica

> **Slow, incomplete inflammation – suppuration and
> scars**

Can expel foreign bodies and promote healing of scar tissue
Ill effects of vaccination
Anxious, sensitive to all impressions. Conscientious about trifles.
Timidity
Sweats. Foot sweat foul
Chronic fistulae and fissures

< cold; air; damp; pressure
> warmth; warm wraps

Spigelia

Violent palpitations

Combined heart and eye symptoms
Violent burning pains like hot needles or wires
Left side
Headache beneath frontal eminence, radiating to eyes
Tongue fissured and coated. Halitosis

◄ tobacco; touch; motion
► lying on right side with head held high; steady pressure;
   3–4 p.m.

Spongia Tosta

> ## Croupy, barking, suffocating cough

Hoarse, dry, burning larynx
Angina. Palpitations. Cannot lie down
Wakes, starting from sleep
Anxiety and fear. Fear of future. Fear of death
Cannot bear tight clothing around trunk

- **<** dry; cold; wind; roused from sleep; exertion
- **>** eating and drinking (especially cough); warm things

Stannum Metallicum

Pains which come and go gradually

Extreme weakness felt in the chest. Marked debility
Mucopurulent secretions from mucous membranes
Feeling of hunger but cannot eat
Nausea or vomiting from odour of cooking food
Anxious, nervous and sad before menses

< motion; using voice; lying on right side; 10 a.m.

> rapid motion; hard pressure over an edge; cough; expectoration

Staphysagria

> ## Ailments from suppressed anger with indignation

Ailments from reproaches; disappointed love; wounded honour
Sexual disturbances and disorders of sexual organs
Cutting, stitching, shooting pains in genitalia
Pain in abdomen after indignation
Craves tobacco, sweets, bread, milk

◀ emotions; indignation; quarrels; touch; cold; lacerations
▶ breakfast; warmth; rest

Sulphur

Chronic inflammation

Redness of orifices. Itchy skin < scratching; washing; at night
Sinking feeling in abdomen about 11 a.m.
Complaints that relapse. When well-indicated remedies fail to act,
especially in acute disease
Hot feet – has to stick them out of bed. Diarrhoea – driving out of
bed in the morning
Lazy, selfish, philosophical, untidy

< suppressions; bathing; becoming overheated; overexertion; milk
> dry, warm weather; open air; motion

Symphytum Officinalis

Promotes healing of broken bones

Bone and periosteal injuries and bruising
Penetrating wounds to perineum and bones
Irritable stump after amputation
Gastric and duodenal ulcers
Externally, as a dressing for sores and pruritus ani

< injuries; blows from blunt instruments; touch
> warmth

Syphylinum

Chronic eruptions and shifting rheumatic pains

Ulceration of mouth, nose, genitals, skin
Succession of abscesses
Depressed. Despairs of recovery. Aversion to company
Utter prostration and debility in the morning
Craves alcohol. Capricious appetite. Aversion to meat

◄ night; sunset to sunrise; damp; during thunderstorms; seashore
► continued or slow motion; applied heat; during day

Thuja Occidentalis

Warts

Ill effects of vaccination
Fixed ideas. Closed. Hurried
Anger from contradiction. Aversion to company
Headache in vertex, as if pierced by a nail
Asthma, when Arsenicum fails to cure, though well indicated

< cold; damp; 3 a.m. and 3 p.m.; onions
> free secretions; sneezing; warmth

Tuberculinum Bovinum

Symptoms
constantly
changing,
well-selected
remedies fail to
improve and cold
is taken from
the least
exposure

> **Symptoms constantly changing, well-selected remedies fail to improve and cold is taken from the least exposure**

Longs for open air. Wants windows open or to ride in a strong wind

Desire to travel

Sensitive to music. Every trifle irritates. Irritability on waking

Children active and precocious mentally, but weak physically

Desire for meat, especially smoked meat, bacon, fat, pork

 close room; exertion; change of weather; damp

▶ cool wind; open air; continued motion

Urtica Urens

Urtica Urens

> **Urticarial eruptions < bathing; warmth; violent exercise**

Urticarial eruptions < bathing; warmth; violent exercise

Antidotes ill effects of eating shellfish
Diminished or absent secretion of breast milk after confinement
Pruritus vulvae with stinging, itching and swelling of parts
Diarrhoea after suppressed eruptions
Gout

< snow-air; yearly; cool moist air; cold bathing
> rubbing; lying down

Veratrum Album

> ## Collapse with extreme coldness, blueness and weakness

Vomiting, purging and cramps in extremities
Postoperative shock with cold perspiration on forehead
Great fainting remedy
Brooding. Haughty. Easily offended. Religious affections
Thirst for cold water, vomited as soon as swallowed

< exertion; drinking; cold drinks; during pain
> warmth; hot drinks; lying

Veratrum Viride

> ## Paroxysmal atrial fibrillation

Sudden, violent conditions
Intense fever with twitching and tendency to spasms
Delirious. Lamenting
Intense congestion. Flushed face
Hiccough. Oesophagitis

< rising; motion; cold
> rubbing; eating; lying with head low

Zincum Metallicum

Tiredness in general

Defective vitality, brain or nerve power
Too weak to develop exanthema, menses, expectoration,
urination, to comprehend or memorize
Changeable moods. Irritability in evening
Torments everyone with his complaints
Restless, fidgety feet

< exhaustion; noise; touch; wine
> free discharges; menses; sweat; motion; appearance of eruptions

GRAPHICS:
COMMUNICATING WITH PATIENTS

'A picture is worth a thousand words' says the old Chinese maxim.

I frequently find a simple pen or pencil drawing helps me to communicate effectively with my patients. Experience has taught me that there are certain drawings which I recreate time and time again.

This section contains those drawings. Each drawing has a short explanatory note attached to it and these notes have been written with the patient as the intended reader.

The drawings can be photocopied for use with your patients and you can scribble on them and let your patients take their own copies home with them, thereby giving them another chance to digest what you had to say to them.

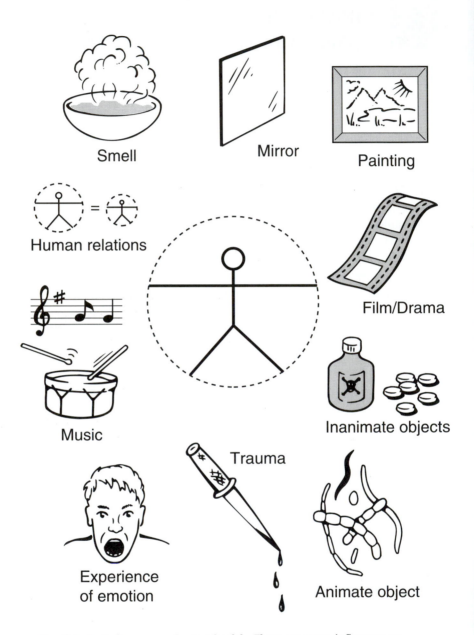

Graphic 1 Influences on human health. There are many influences on human health and not all of them involve molecules. This illustration shows some of the possible influences which include music, emotion and visual images.

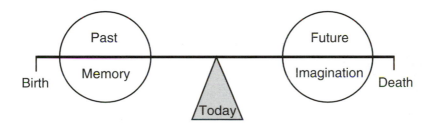

Graphic 2 People are often paralysed by either their traumatic memories of the past, or their overwhelming fears of the future. In fact, we are only truly alive in the present moment – *today*. The time-line of a life, illustrated here, shows that the past exists only in our memory and that the future exists only in our imaginations. Only today is real.

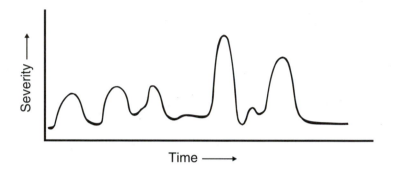

Graphic 3a All chronic diseases demonstrate a pattern of relapses and remissions. This graph shows this basic pattern of 'flare-ups' and 'good spells'.

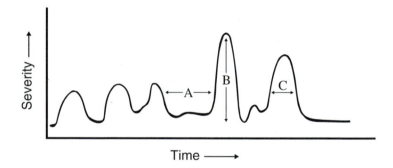

Graphic 3b Linked to the previous graph (Graphic 3a), this graphic helps to illustrate the aims of treatment in the management of chronic disease. We aim to achieve three goals: A. Increase the distance between 'flare-ups' (or relapses); B. Decrease the severity of 'flare-ups'; C. Decrease the duration of 'flare-ups'.

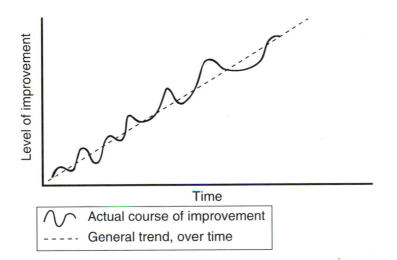

Graphic 4 Following on from Graphics 3a and b, this graph illustrates the concept that improvement in a chronic condition will not be without setbacks. Every day will not necessarily be better than any previous day.

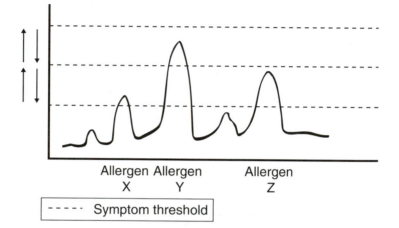

Allergen X   Allergen Y   Allergen Z

- - - - - Symptom threshold

Graphic 5   There are two main ways to tackle the problem of allergies, homeopathically. Either by treating individual allergies, e.g. with nosodes of the allergens, or by making a 'constitutional' prescription to reduce the overall sensitivity to allergens in the patient. This graph helps to demonstrate this. Most people who suffer allergies are sensitive to more than one allergen. The particular allergens which cause symptoms apparently vary. The peaks on the graph represent one individual's response to different allergens – x, y and z. The dotted line represents a symptom 'threshold' below which the allergens do not manifest symptoms. Treatment can be aimed at raising the threshold by using a well-chosen constitutional remedy.

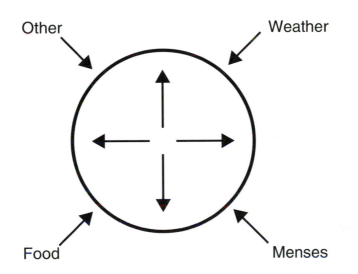

Graphic 6   Why have I become ill? Illnesses are usually the result of a
combination of many factors. Some factors affect us from outside our bodies
and some are the result of changes in levels of vitamins, minerals, hormones,
etc inside our bodies.

GRAPHICS

APPENDIX – MIASMS

The subject of miasms is too detailed to describe fully in this book. It is, however, a significant part of Hahnemann's medical philosophy and certainly of his understanding of chronic disease.

I have asked many of the leading contemporary homeopaths whether or not they find these ideas of practical use. Unanimously, they say they seldom employ such concepts in their daily work. Prescribing on the basis of miasms is, apparently, not so common, unless the miasmatic remedy chosen fits the case well in terms of totality – which is really another prescribing strategy.

However, what is a miasm? A miasm is postulated to be either an inherited or an acquired condition which predisposes the patient to a chronic disease. Hahnemann originally described three miasms – Psora, Syphilis and Sycosis (Gonorrhoea) – and suggested that they were at the root of all chronic disease. The idea has been extended with the evolution of medical knowledge. Tuberculosis is also now thought to have a miasmatic influence. Indeed, a look at the 'ailments from' or 'never well since' rubrics of the Repertory will give you an idea about the possible range of miasms.

Clinically, a prescriber may think of a miasm when dealing with a chronic condition with a strong family history. Eczema presenting virtually from birth in a child with a strong family history of eczema may hint, for example, at the psoric miasm.

Each of the miasms has a nosode associated with it which is used in the treatment of the condition. The nosodes are as follows:

- Psora – Psorinum
- Syphilis – Syphilinum (otherwise known as Lueticum)
- Sycosis – Medorrhinum
- Tuberculosis – Tuberculinum.

Hahnemann went on to develop this theory and classified remedies according to their shared features of the various miasms. You may therefore hear homeopaths talk about a psoric remedy, e.g. Sulphur. Some prescribers even consciously make an assessment of the relative influences of the various miasms in any particular case. Prescribers using miasmatic approaches may give the miasmatic remedy first, then follow up with a similimum or may use the miasmatic remedy intercurrently.

I will not detail the features of the miasmatic nosodes here but refer the reader to other texts. Koehler's book (see Bibliography) has a good introduction to this subject, but all the main materia medicae contain descriptions of these nosodes. Suffice it to say that Psora is the itch disease with skin complaints and allergies, Sycosis has a strong feature of irritability, restlessness and inflammation (especially urogenital) and Syphilis has destructive and degenerative processes.

GLOSSARY

Aggravation. An initial, temporary worsening of existing symptoms. An aggravation is usually considered a good prognostic indicator.

Autonosode. A nosode prepared from tissue of the individual to whom the remedy is to be given.

Isopathy. Treatment of an allergic condition with a homeopathically prepared remedy made from the provoking allergen.

Materia medica. A list of remedies with associated descriptions of their characteristics, the source material being obtained from provings, toxicology and cured cases.

Miasms. Postulated basis of chronic disease. Either acquired or inherited.

Modality. A modifying factor which affects a symptom. Commonly accepted shorthand is < meaning 'aggravating factor' and > meaning 'ameliorating factor'.

Mother tincture. The original substance dissolved in alcohol, but undiluted.

Nosodes. Remedies prepared from disease products, diseased tissue or pathogens, for example, Tuberculinum Bovinum, Herpes Zoster nosode and glandular fever nosode.

Polychrest. A well-known remedy with a wide applicability based on a wide-ranging symptom picture.

Potency. The strength of the remedy. Decimal scale, denoted by X or D is a series of 1:9 dilutions and succussions. Centessimal scale, denoted by C is a series of 1:99 dilutions and succussions. LM scale is a 1 in 50 000 dilution series used by Hahnemann.

Proving. Testing of a substance on healthy volunteers.

Repertory. An encyclopaedia of symptoms arranged in a particular order (usually one chapter per body system), with associated lists of remedies which have these symptoms as part of their characteristic picture.

Similimum. The single remedy which best matches the symptoms of the patient.

Succussion. Vigorous shaking of the solution at each stage of dilution.

Tautopathy. Treatment of a condition using a remedy prepared from a pharmaceutical drug.

Trituration. The process of grindling an insoluble substance with lactose powder to obtain a soluble substance for the preparation of a remedy.

BIBLIOGRAPHY

Articles

Anderson E, Anderson P 1987 General practitioners and alternative medicine. Journal of Royal College of General Practitioners 37:52–55

Brigo, Serpelloni G 1991 Homoeopathic treatment of migraines. A randomised double blind controlled study of sixty cases. Berlin Journal of Research in Homoeopathy 1 (2):98

Dorfman P, Lasserre M, Tetau M 1987 Preparation a l'acouchement par homoeopathie. Experimentation en double insu versus placebo. Cahiers Biotherapie 94:77

Ferley J P, et al 1989 A controlled evaluation of a homoeopathic preparation in influenza-like syndromes. British Journal of Clinical Pharmacology 27:329

Fisher P, et al 1989 Effect of homoeopathic treatment on fibrositis. British Medical Journal 299:365

Gibson R G, et al 1980 Homoeopathic therapy I. Rheumatoid arthritis: evaluation by double blind clinical therapeutic trial. British Journal of Clinical Pharmacology 9:453

Jacobs J, et al 1994 Treatment of acute childhood diarrhoea with homoeopathic medicine: a randomised clinical trial in Nicaragua. Paediatrics 93:719

Kleijnen J, Knipschild P 1991 Clinical trials of homoeopathy. British Medical Journal 302:316

Osler 1892 Principles and practices of medicine.

Reilly D, et al 1994 Is evidence for homoeopathy reproducible? Lancet 344:1601

Taylor Reilly D, et al 1986 Is homoeopathy a placebo response? Lancet 2:881

Books

Bellavite P, Signorini A 1995 Homoeopathy – a frontier in medical science. North Atlantic Books, Berkeley

Boericke W 1987 Homoeopathic materia medica. Homoeopathic Book Service, London

Boger C M 1900 A synoptic key of the materia medica. Indian Books and Periodical Syndicate, New Delhi

Boyd H 1989 Introduction to homoeopathic medicine. Beaconsfield Publishers, Beaconsfield, UK

Gibson D 1987 Studies of homoeopathic remedies. Beaconsfield Publishers, Beaconsfield, UK

Hahnemann H 1986 Organon of medicine, 6th edn (translated by Kunzli J) Gollancz, London

Koehler G 1986 The handbook of homoeopathy. Thorsons, Wellingborough, Northamptonshire, UK

Kuhn T 1962 The structure of scientific revolutions. University of Chicago Press, Chicago

Nash E 1988 Leaders in homoeopathic therapeutics. Jain, New Delhi

Phatak S 1988 Materia medica of homoeopathic medicines. Foxlee-Vaughan, London

Scholten J 1993 Homeopathy and minerals. Stichting Alonnissos, Utrecht

Scholten J 1996 Homeopathy and the elements. Stichting Alonnissos, Utrecht

Schroyens, F (ed) 1993 Synthesis. Repertorium homoeopathicum syntheticum edited by Homoeopathic Book Publishers and Archibel SA, London

Vermeulen F 1992 Synoptic materia medica. Merlijn, Harlem

Vermeulen F 1994 Concordant materia medica. Merlijn, Harlem

Vithoulkas G 1986 The science of homoeopathy. ASOHM, Athens

Von Lippe A 1988 Key notes and red line symptoms of materia medica. Jain, New Delhi

INDEX

Carbo Vegetalis, **168**
Carcinosin, **169**
    family history of cancer, 169
    nightmares/night terrors, 110
Cardiac dilation, 181
Case record sheets, 45, 46–48, 78
Catarrh, 158, 184, 229
    eustachian, 194
    hoarseness, 141
    recurrent, 112
    see also Nasal discharge
Caulophyllum, **170**
    labour ,15, 119, 170
Causticum, **171**
    grief, 100, 171
    osteoarthritis, 126
    urinary incontinence with cough,
       171
    warts, 116
Centesimal scale of potentization, 16, 17,
    31
Central disturbances, 50
Centre of gravity, 50, 58
Cervical dystocia, 21
Chamomilla, **172**
    teething problems, 113, 172
Chelidonium Majus, **173**
    gall bladder colic, 98
    right–sided symptoms, 173
Chickenpox, 94
Childhood problems, 118
    colic, 96
    enuresis, 118
    headache with diarrhoea, 163
    measles, 108
    mumps, 109
    nose picking, 176
    teething, 113
    tooth grinding, 176
    see also Catarrh
Chillblains, 95
China Officinalis, **174**
    debility from fluid loss, 174
    tinnitus, 114
Chronic disease, 5, 6–7, 32, 53
    bowel nosodes, 159
    dosing frequency, 61
    follow–up appointments, 75
    graphics, 255–261
    length of consultation, 74
    miasms, 58–59, 263–264
Cimicifuga Racemosa, **175**
    dysfunctional labour, 119, 175

Cina, **176**
'Classical' homeopathy, 29
Clinical
    compendia, 79
    experience, 21–22
    research, 19–21, 27
Clumsiness, 140
Cocculus, **177**
Coffea Cruda, **178**
Cognitive function, 43
Cold
    intolerance, 200, 211
    sensitivity to, 140
Coldness, 163, 182
    local, 225
    sexual organs, 166
Colic, 96, 172, 179, 209, 226
    during and after menses, 203
Collapse, 252
Colleagues
    dealing with, 83–85
    referrals from, 35–36
    support from seniors, 85
Colocynthis, **179**, 15
    colic, 96, 179
    dysmenorrhoea, 130
    neuralgias, 133
Common questions *see* Questions,
    common
Company, 43
Complementary medicine, 4
    doctors' attitudes to, 4–5
    homeopathy as, 5–6
The Complete Repertory, 53
Complete symptoms, 45, 51
Complexiste school, 29–30
Computer repertories, 55
    using, 57–58
Confidence, lack of, 208
Confrontation, 43
Confusion, 153, 184, 190
    of identity, 143
    while walking, 221
Congestion, 159
Conium, **180**
    impotence, 101
    indurations in breasts, 180
    mastalgia, 107
Conjunctivitis, 229
Consolation, 43
Constipation, 128, 143, 226
Constriction, sensations of, 161
Consultant colleagues, 84

Indications for homeopathy, 87–134
  no effective allopathic treatment,
      91–116
  reduction of allopathic treatment,
      127–134
  unacceptable side-effect profile,
      122–126
  unsafe for allopathic treatment,
      117–121
  well established, 36
Indifference, colleague, 84
Infant snuffles, 102, 144, 199, 237
Infertility, 103, 158
Inflammation, chronic, 246
Influenza, 104, 189
  see also Flu-like illness,
      Oscillococcinum trial
Influenzinum, 104
Information
  leaflets, 82
  paradigm of, 23–26
Injuries, 105, 150
  broken bones, 247
  bruising, 105, 150, 231, 234
  crush injuries, 105, 133, 195
  deep trauma or septic wounds, 156
  penetrating wounds, 247
  puncture wounds, 105, 195, 206
  tendon and ligament, 105, 234
  torn or ragged wounds, 165
Insect bites, 206
Insomnia, 181
  nervous sleeplessness, 178
Integration of homeopathy
  appointments into routine practice,
      76
  history into case notes, 77
  into primary care team, 73–74
Intellectual achievement, physician's,
      8–9
Intermittent claudication, 106, 161
Introduction to daily practice, 3
Involuntary movements, 140
Iodum, **197**
Ipecacuanha, **198**, 120
Isopathy, 59–60, 91, 265
Itching, 145, 213, 228, 233, 246

J

Jaundice, 98, 173, 238
Jealousy, 43, 148, 205

K

Kali Bichromum, **199**
  migrating pain, 199
  recurrent catarrh, 112
Kali Carbonicum, **200**
  asthma, 127
  backache and weakness, 200
Kali Phosphoricum, **201**
Kali Sulphuricum, **202**
Kent's Repertory, 53, 54
Keynotes, 52, 58, 137
  premenstrual syndrome, 16
Korsakoff, single vial method, 17
Krebiozen ,25
  placebo response, 26
Kreosotum, **203**

L

Labour ,15, 119, 170, 175
  trial of remedies, 21
Lac caninum, **204**
Lachesis, **205**, 59
  jealousy, 205
  premenstrual syndrome, 15–16, 111
Lactose delivery agents, 17
The Lancet, 20
Ledum, **206**
  puncture wounds, 105
'Lifelines', 26
Ligament injuries, 105
Lilium Tigrinum, **207**
Limbs, aching, 230
Lips, white, 187
Liver disease, 173
LM scale of potentization, 17
Local symptoms, 40, 50
Localization, sensation, 39
Loquacity, 205, 227
Lothian Health pilot homeopathic clinic, 5
Low potency, 31
Lung infection, right, 173
Lycopodium, **208**
  anticipatory anxiety, 117
  flatulent dyspepsia, 208
  impotence, 101

M

Magnesia Phosphorica, **209**

Magnesia Phosphorica (*contd*)
  colic, 96
  dysmenorrhoea, 209
Magnesium Phosphoricum, 130
Malaria, 12
Malnutrition, 159
Mangialavori, Massimo, 60
Margins, recording history, 44–45, 77
Mastalgia, 107
Mastitis, 224
Materia Medica, 22, 23, 52, 53, 79,
        135–254, 265
Measles, 108
Medication *see* Allopathic drugs
Medorrhinum, **263**
  asthma, 210
Memory problems, 143, 145
Menses
  amenorrhoea, 186
  bright red with nausea, 198
  dysmenorrhoea, 103, 130, 186, 209
  flow only when moving about, 207
  frequent, 188
  irregular heavy, 239
  metrorrhagia, 192
Menstrual history, 42
Mental
  disturbances, 50
    see also Anxiety; Confusion;
        Depression; Mood
  slowness, 154
  state examination, 42–44
Mercurius Corrosivus, **212**
Mercurius (Merc Sol), **211**
  cold/heat intolerance, 211
  influenza, 104
  mumps, 109
  teething problems, 113
Metrorrhagia, 192
Mezereum, **213**
  chickenpox, 94
  shingles, 213
Miasms, 58–59, 263–264, 265
Mid potency, 31
Migraine, 51, 132, 215, 238
  trial of homeopathic remedies, 21
Minimum effective dose, 12–13
Miscarriage, 167
  threatened, 236
Modalities, 39–40, 41, 42, 265
Molecular biology, 23, 24, 27
Mood
  changeability of, 187, 196, 254

  sentimental, 146
Morgan Co., **159**
Mother tincture, 16, 17, 18, 265
Mouth, dry, 201
Movements, exaggerated, 140
Mucous membranes
  dryness, 160
  irritation, 159
  mucopurulent secretions, 244
  sticky secretions, 233
Mucus
  from throat and rectum, 142
  rattling, 147, 164, 202
Multiple vial method, 17
Mumps, 109, 224
Murphy's Repertory, 53
Muscles, sore, 153, 156

N

Naloxone, 26
Nasal discharge, 186, 214, 238
  excoriating, 91, 141
  see also Catarrh
Nasal polyps, 238
Natrum Carbonicum, **214**
Natrum Muriaticum, **215**
  anxiety, 123
  grief, 100, 215
  infertility, 103
  migraine, 132
Natrum Phosphoricum, **216**
Natrum Sulphuricum, **217**
  asthma, 127
  head injury, mental ill effects, 217
Nature, 26
Nausea, 147, 219, 221, 244
  continuous, 198
  pregnancy, 120
  travel sickness, 177
Nerve injuries, 156
Nervous
  sleeplessness, 178
  tension, 159
Neuralgias, 133, 161, 179, 226
Night
  cramps, 125
  sweats, 174
Nightmares/night terrors, 110
Nipple
  pain, 107
  retracted, 194

INDEX

Trembling, 147, 175, 216
Trials *see* Randomized clinical trials
Trituration, 16, 18, 266
Tuberculinum, 263
Tuberculinum Bovinum, **250**
Tuberculosis, 263
Twitching and spasms, 176, 220, 239
Typefaces and strengths, 55, 56

U

Ulcerations, 211, 248
Ulcers, 199
    gastric and duodenal, 247
Underlining, recording symptoms, 44, 45, 77
The Uniciste school, 29
Urethral syndrome, 115, 167
Urgency, 167
    stool, 142, 212
    urinary, 179, 203
        see also Cystitis
Urinary incontinence, 171, 203
Urination
    copious amounts, 222
    starting and stopping, 180
    see also Cystitis
Urine
    difficulty in passing, 148
    retention after confinement, 220
Urtica Urens, 91, **251**
Urticaria, 91, 184, 232, 251

V

Vaccination ill effects, 241, 249
Vaginal
    dryness, 103
    prolapse, 227
Vaginismus, 157
Varicose veins, 156, 192
Venous
    circulation, 207
    congestion, 188

stasis, 156
Veratrum Album, **252**
    collapse, 252
    night cramps, 125
Veratum Viride, **253**
Vertigo, 158, 180, 219
Vesicles, 232
    bluish, 231
Vomiting, 147, 185, 188, 252
    bile, 238
    from cooking food odour, 244
    pregnancy, 118
    relieved by cold water, 182
    sour, 216

W

Warts, 116, 249
Waterbrash, 221
Weakness, 144, 147, 152, 168, 181, 235
    tiredness in general, 254
    mental, then physical, 222
    of muscles, heart and intellect, 200
Weather, 41–42
Weepy, 229
Weighting symptoms, 44, 57
Whooping cough, 183
World Journal of Surgery, 25
Wrong
    potency, 65
    remedy, 63

Y

The Yellow Emperor's Classic of Medicine, 37

Z

Zincum Metallicum, **254**
    chillblains, 95
    tiredness in general, 254